Staff Library
Singleton Hospital
Tel: 0170? · ?8? · Ex? 5?8?

# Nutritional Strategies for the Very Low Birthweight Infant

# WITHDRAWN

**Singleton Staff Library**
*S007264*

# Nutritional Strategies for the Very Low Birthweight Infant

David H. Adamkin

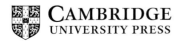

CAMBRIDGE
UNIVERSITY PRESS

CAMBRIDGE UNIVERSITY PRESS
Cambridge, New York, Melbourne, Madrid, Cape Town, Singapore,
São Paulo, Delhi, Dubai, Tokyo

Cambridge University Press
The Edinburgh Building, Cambridge CB2 8RU, UK

Published in the United States of America by Cambridge
University Press, New York

www.cambridge.org
Information on this title: www.cambridge.org/9780521732468

© D. H. Adamkin 2009

This publication is in copyright. Subject to statutory exception
and to the provisions of relevant collective licensing agreements,
no reproduction of any part may take place without
the written permission of Cambridge University Press.

First published 2009

Printed in the United Kingdom at the University Press, Cambridge

*A catalogue record for this publication is available from the British Library*

*Library of Congress Cataloguing in Publication data*
Adamkin, David H.
   Nutritional strategies for the very low birthweight infant / David H. Adamkin.
      p.   cm.
   Includes bibliographical references and index.
   ISBN 978-0-521-73246-8
   1. Birth weight, Low–Diet therapy.   2. Premature infants–Nutrition.   I. Title.
   RJ281.A335   2009
   618.92′011–dc22         2009024647

ISBN 978-0-521-73246-8 paperback

Cambridge University Press has no responsibility for the persistence or
accuracy of URLs for external or third-party internet websites referred to
in this publication, and does not guarantee that any content on such
websites is, or will remain, accurate or appropriate.

Every effort has been made in preparing this publication to provide
accurate and up-to-date information which is in accord with accepted
standards and practice at the time of publication. Although case histories
are drawn from actual cases, every effort has been made to disguise the
identities of the individuals involved. Nevertheless, the authors, editors
and publishers can make no warranties that the information contained
herein is totally free from error, not least because clinical standards are
constantly changing through research and regulation. The authors, editors
and publishers therefore disclaim all liability for direct or consequential
damages resulting from the use of material contained in this publication.
Readers are strongly advised to pay careful attention to information provided
by the manufacturer of any drugs or equipment that they plan to use.

*This book is dedicated to my partner in both Academics and life, my wife, Carol. Also to our children Stephanie, Michelle and Matthew, who have all chosen medical careers, dedicating their lives to the care of others.*

# CONTENTS

# ACKNOWLEDGEMENT

I am grateful to be blessed by the work and talent of three wonderful people and dear friends who have reviewed and contributed sections to this manuscript: Deborah Abel, Jatinder Bhatia and Gilbert Martin. Their input is greatly appreciated.

## The following expert neonatologists assisted Professor Adamkin in the preparation of this book

### Dr. Gilbert Martin, MD

Dr. Martin is Director Emeritus of the Neonatal Intensive Care Unit at Citrus Valley Medical Center in West Covina, California. He is a Clinical Professor of Pediatrics at the University of California (Irvine), and the University of Southern California. He is Editor Emeritus of the Journal of Perinatology. He is the Chairman of the Coding Training Committee for the American Academy of Pediatrics, Section of Perinatal Pediatrics. He is a member of the Committee of Practice Management, a past member of the Committee of the Fetus and Newborn and a member of the Executive Committee of the Perinatal Section. He is past-president of the California Perinatal Association,

the California Association of Neonatologists, co-chair
of the Neoprep Committee and a member of the Pediatrix
Medical Group.

### Dr. Jatinder Bhatia, MD

Dr. Bhatia is Professor and Chief of the Section of Neonatology,
Department of Pediatrics at the Medical College of Georgia in
Augusta, Georgia, USA. He is also an honorary consultant for
Philippine Children's Medical Center in Quezon City. He is a
recipient of the Distinguished Faculty Award for Institutional
Service at the Medical College of Georgia and the Georgia
Nutrition Council Award of Excellence. He is also secretary-
treasurer for the Southern Society of Pediatric Research
and was recently appointed to the American Academy of
Pediatrics Committee of Nutrition. He is a member of the
Society for Pediatric Research, the American Pediatric Society,
the American Institute of Nutrition, the American Society for
Clinical Nutrition, the American Society for Parenteral and
Enteral Nutrition, the American Academy of Pediatrics and the
American Dietetic Association.

### Professor Adamkin was also assisted by

### Deborah Abel, MS, RD

Deborah Abel is a Visiting Lecturer and Coordinator for the
Leadership in MCH Nutrition Program, Indiana University
School of Health and Rehabilitation Sciences, and, Neonatal-
Pediatric Dietitian for James Whitcomb Riley Hospital

for Children at the Indiana University Medical Center, Indianapolis, IN. The Leadership in MCH Nutrition Program is a nationally recognized program whose mission is to improve the nutrition, health and well-being of high-risk and vulnerable infants and children through the education of pediatric nutrition fellows, graduate students who are dietitians and other health care professionals in Indiana and beyond. Additionally, the MCH Nutrition program provides leadership and pediatric nutrition education for the MCH Nutrition provider community, online pediatric nutrition education modules for continuing education nationally, and consultation nationally and regionally as leaders in the field of pediatric nutrition. Ms. Abel has had a key role in developing and delivering the course entitled "Nutrition for the High Risk Infant in Intensive Care and Following Discharge" and other modules for the e-learning graduate/professional certificate program "Leadership in Clinical Pediatric Nutrition." She is completing a doctoral program in Health and Rehabilitation Sciences (Pediatric Nutrition Emphasis), Indiana University.

SINGLETON HOSPITAL
STAFF LIBRARY

# FOREWORD

Neonatology as a subspecialty was established in 1975. There have been adventures and misadventures. There have been advances and declines. However, with a greater understanding of normal development and physiology, the improvements in technology and the utilization of evidence-based medicine, our subspecialty continues to thrive. Much of our success has been due to the better use of ventilation techniques and the development of newer antibiotics to treat infectious conditions.

However, it was known early on that nutrition was an essential part of our equation for success. With the increasing survival of premature and extremely premature infants and the increasing incidence of prematurity, nutrition as an adjunct to the care of the tiny premature infant is of paramount importance. Appropriate nutritional therapy should allow for maximum growth without adverse effects and evidence suggests that infants who grow at the highest quartiles have better neurocognitive outcomes. It is also well recognized that extrauterine growth restriction due to other morbidities and inadequate nutritional intervention can lead to poor outcomes. The full-term infant and late-preterm infant have multiple avenues available to provide adequate nutrition for growth. However, the preterm and especially the extremely low birthweight infant (ELBW) still present great challenges.

This monograph entitled "Nutritional Strategies for the Very Low Birthweight Infant" presents a method to understand the complexity of nutrition in this gestational age and weight group and to provide "strategies" for therapy. The chapters discuss energy, the basic components of nutrition (carbohydrate, protein, fat), vitamins, minerals and trace elements. In addition, there is information regarding human milk, infant formulas and influences on neurodevelopmental and growth outcomes. Each chapter provides the reader with recommendations and guidelines for therapy. This monograph is intended for the caregiver of a neonate, from a medical student or dietitian to the advance practice nurse and neonatologist. The material presented is based on evidence for best practice and provides guidelines for nutritional intervention in this very vulnerable group of neonates.

Gilbert I. Martin, MD
Jatinder Bhatia, MD

# GLOSSARY

| | |
|---|---|
| ARA | arachidonic acid |
| BPD | bronchopulmonary dysplasia |
| CPAP | continuous positive airway pressure |
| DBM | donor breast milk |
| DHA | docosahexanoic acid |
| ECW | extracellular water |
| EFAD | essential fatty acids deficiency |
| ELBW | infant birthweight $\leq 1000$ g |
| FFA/ALB | free fatty acid: albumin ratio |
| FFA | free fatty acids |
| GIR | glucose infusion rate |
| GRV | gastric residual volume |
| ICW | intracellular water |
| IUGR | intrauterine growth restriction |
| IVL | intravenous lipid |
| MEN | minimal enteral nutrition |
| NEC | necrotizing enterocolitis |
| NPC | nonprotein calories |
| PDA | patent ductus arteriosis |
| PDF | post-discharge formula |
| PNAC | parenteral nutrition-associated cholestasis |
| PPHN | persistent pulmonary hypertension |

| | |
|---|---|
| PTF | preterm formula |
| PUFA | polyunsaturated fatty acids |
| RMR | resting metabolic rate |
| RTBW | return to birthweight |
| SGA | small for gestational age |
| TBW | total body water |
| TF | term formula |
| TPN | total parenteral nutrition |
| TPNAC | total parenteral nutrition-associated cholestasis |
| UAC | umbilical artery catheterization |
| VLBW | infant birthweight $\leq 1500$ g |

# Chapter 1

# Introduction

This book provides a clinical practicum to implement parenteral and enteral feeding guidelines for aggressive nutrition to prevent extrauterine growth failure of the very low birthweight (VLBW), ≤1500 gram infant. These strategies promote the goals of reducing postnatal weight loss, earlier return to birthweight, and improved catch-up growth. The guiding principle for these strategies is that undernutrition is, by definition, non-physiologic and undesirable. It follows that any measure that diminishes undernutrition is inherently good provided that safety is not compromised. Further, this book will review available evidence concerning the controversy of rapid early growth leading to visceral adiposity and metabolic/cardiovascular morbidity in adolescence and adulthood.

Although current guidelines for the growth of preterm infants use intrauterine growth as the reference standard, the growth of most preterm and VLBW infants proceeds at a slower rate than in utero. Although many of the smallest VLBW infants are also born small for gestational age (SGA), both appropriate-for-gestational-age VLBW and SGA infants develop extrauterine growth restriction. Figure 1.1, from the National Institute of Child Health and Human Development

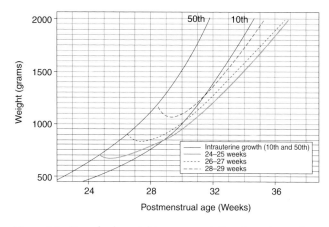

Figure 1.1. Mean body weight versus gestational age in weeks for all study infants who had gestational ages at birth between 24 and 29 weeks. Reference: Ehrenkranz RA, et al. *Pediatrics* 1999; 104:280–289. Reproduced with permission.

(NICHD) Neonatal Research Network, demonstrates the differences between intrauterine growth and the observed rates of postnatal growth in the NICHD study. The postnatal growth curves are shifted to the right of the reference curves in each gestational age category. This "growth deficiency" is common in extremely low birthweight (ELBW) infants (≤1000 gram birthweight).

Figure 1.2 shows three nutritional strategies, in the boxes, superimposed on the NICHD growth observation study. Figure 1.3 is a nutritional "map" for the VLBW infant including a time-line configuration in which the boxes arbitrarily divide nutritional management into three segments beginning at birth and continuing for 9–12 months corrected age.

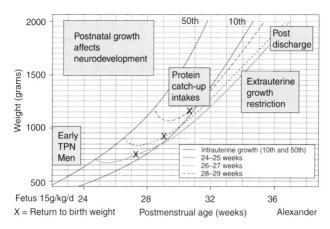

Figure 1.2. NICHD Growth Observational Study. Adapted from Ehrenkranz RA, et al. *Pediatrics* 1999; 104:280–289. Reproduced with permission.

As shown in Figure 1.2, optimizing neurodevelopment is the ultimate goal of promoting growth in the neonatal intensive care unit. Considerable evidence suggests that early growth deficits have long-lasting consequences, including short stature and poor neurodevelopmental outcomes. The most convincing data concerning the neurodevelopmental consequences of inadequate early nutrition are those reported in studies by Lucas and Ehrenkranz. Lucas demonstrated that preterm infants fed a preterm formula containing a higher content of protein and other nutrients over the first postnatal month had higher neurodevelopmental indices at both 18 months and seven to eight years of age compared with preterm infants fed term formula. Ehrenkranz examined (Chapter 23) the relationship between growth in the neonatal intensive

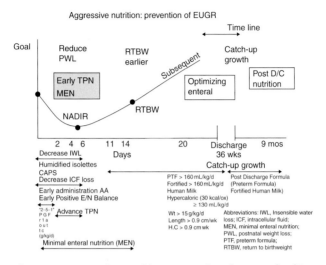

**Figure 1.3. Aggressive nutrition: Prevention of EUGR.** Adamkin DH. Feeding the preterm infant. In: J Bhatia, ed. *Perinatal Nutrition Optimizing Infant Health and Development.* New York, NY: Marcel Dekker; 2004: 165–190. Reproduced with permission.

care unit and later neurodevelopment and growth outcomes. The study demonstrated improved developmental and growth outcomes at 18 to 22 months of age for ELBW infants who had higher growth velocities for weight and head circumference during the neonatal intensive care unit hospitalization. As elusive as is the goal for VLBW infants that nutrition should support "postnatal growth" approximating in utero fetal growth, the fetal model is sound and there is no alternative model or "gold standard."

The goal of nutritional management in VLBW infants, which is supported by the American Academy of Pediatrics

Committee on Nutrition, is the achievement of postnatal growth at a rate that approximates the intrauterine growth of a normal fetus at the same postconceptional age. In reality, however, the growth of VLBW infants lags considerably after birth. Such infants, especially those weighing less than 1000 g at birth (ELBW), typically do not regain birthweight until two to three weeks of age.

Nutrient intakes of VLBW infants are much lower than the nutrient intake that the fetus receives in utero. This intake deficit often persists throughout much of the infants' hospital stay. Although non-nutritional factors (morbidities) are involved in the slow growth of VLBW infants, nutrient deficiencies are critical in explaining delayed growth.

Neu and colleagues have recently suggested goals that are more meaningful than just somatic growth. These include:

- Maintenance of lean body mass and bone density
- Prevention of complications (e.g. chronic lung disease, necrotizing enterocolitis, and infection)
- Optimization of neurodevelopment
- Adult health

We address nutritional practices in this book and try to examine not only nutrient balance and growth but also the impact on neurodevelopment and health outcomes.

Evidence and experience often dictates the neonatologist's approach to patient care. Ehrenkranz recently reviewed the strength of the evidence for common nutritional practices for VLBW infants. Table 1.1, adapted from an AAP steering committee in a policy statement, weighs the quality of the

**Table 1.1.** Evidence-based early nutritional practice for VLBW infants: recommendations and evidence quality

| Practice | Strength of recommendation[a] | Evidence quality[b] |
|---|---|---|
| **Prompt provision of energy:** Glucose infusion providing about 6 mg/kg/min Increase to about 10 mg/kg/d by 7 days of life Maintain blood sugar 50–120 mg/dL | Recommended | B |
| **Prompt provision of parenteral amino acids:** Initiate 3.0 g/kg/d within hours of birth Advance to 4.0 g/kg/d by 0.5–1.0 g/kg/d steps | Recommended | B |
| **Initiate lipid emulsion within the first 24–30 hrs of birth:** Start 0.5–1.0 g/kg/d Advance to 3.0–3.5 g/kg/d by 0.5–1.0g/kg/d steps | Recommended | B |
| **Initiate trophic feedings by 5 days of age:** Provide about 10 mL/kg/d (human milk if possible) Begin advancing to ~150 mL/kg/d by 10–20 mL/kg/d steps within the next several days | Recommended | B |

Adapted with permission from the AAP Steering Committee on Quality Improvement and Management: Marcuse EK, Shiffman RN. Classifying recommendations for clinical practice guidelines. *Pediatrics* 2004; 114: 874–877.

[a] Strength of recommendation: strongly recommended; recommended; option; not recommended

[b] Evidence quality: A, well-designed, RCTs performed on appropriate populations; B, RCTs with minor limitations, overwhelmingly consistent evidence from observational studies;

C, observational studies (case-control and cohort design);

D, expert opinion (case reports, reasoning from first principles).

evidence for practices and strategies utilized in clinical neonatology.

We have followed this evidence-based information in writing this monograph.

## SUGGESTED READING

Adamkin DH. Feeding the preterm infant. In: J Bhatia, ed. *Perinatal Nutrition Optimizing Infant Health and Development.* New York: Marcel Dekker; 2004:165–190.

Ehrenkranz RA. Early, aggressive nutritional management for very low birth weight infants: what is the evidence? *Semin Perinatol* 2007; **31**:48–55.

Ehrenkranz RA, Younes N, Lemons J, et al. Longitudinal growth of hospitalized very-low-birth-weight infants. *Pediatrics* 1999; **104**:280–289.

Kleinman RE (ed). Nutritional needs of the preterm infant. In: *Pediatric Nutrition Handbook*, 5th ed. Elk Grove Village, IL: American Academy of Pediatrics; 2004:23–54.

Lucas A, Morley R, Cole TJ. Randomised trial of early diet in preterm babies and later intelligence quotient. *BMJ* 1998; **317**:1481–148.

The AAP Steering Committee on Quality Improvement and Management: Marcuse EK, Shiffman RN. Classifying recommendations for clinical practice guidelines. Policy statement. *Pediatrics* 2004; **114**:874–877.

# Chapter 2

# Fluid and electrolyte management (Na, Cl and K)

The 24-week fetus is composed of 90% total body water (TBW). Cell membranes separate intracellular water and extracellular water spaces. Sixty-five percent of TBW is in the extracellular (ECW) compartment and 25% is intracellular (ICW). As gestation proceeds towards term, TBW decreases to 74% of total body weight and the extracellular and intracellular volumes are 40% and 35%, respectively. Potassium ($K^+$) is the major ion of the ICW and potassium's intracellular concentration is impaired by insufficient supplies of oxygen and energy. The major ion of ECW is sodium ($Na^+$) and the major anion is chloride ($Cl^-$).

The preterm infant is in a state of relative extracellular fluid volume with an excess of TBW compared with the full-term infant. VLBW infants are vulnerable to imbalances between intra- and extracellular compartments. The dilute urine and negative sodium balance the first few days after birth in the preterm infant is an appropriate adaptive response to extrauterine life. Therefore, the initial diuresis is physiologic, reflecting changes in interstitial fluid volume. This diuresis should be considered in the estimation of daily fluid needs. As a result, a gradual weight loss of 10–15% in a VLBW infant during the first week of life is expected without adversely affecting urine output, urine osmolality, or clinical status. Provision of large volumes of fluid to provide increased nutrition, for example, 160 to 180 mL/kg/d, does not prevent this weight loss and appears to increase the risk of the development of patent ductus arteriosus, intraventricular hemorrhage, bronchopulmonary dysplasia (BPD), and necrotizing enterocolitis (NEC). Therefore, a careful and conservative approach to fluid and nutritional management is appropriate. It appears that the preterm infant can adjust water excretion within a relatively broad range of fluid intake (65–70 mL/kg/d to 140 mL/kg/d) without disturbing renal concentrating abilities or electrolyte balance.

Estimation of daily fluid requirements includes insensible water losses (IWL) from the respiratory tract and skin, gastrointestinal losses (emesis, ostomy output, diarrhea), urinary losses, and losses from drainage catheters (chest tubes). IWL is a passive process and is not regulated by the infant. However, the environmental conditions in which the infant is nursed should be controlled to minimize losses (Table 2.1).

The transepithelial losses are dependent on gestational age, the thickness of the skin and stratum corneum, and blood flow to the skin. The preterm infant has a large body surface area to body weight ratio, with thinner, highly vascularized, more permeable skin. These factors increase heat and fluid losses, and placing a cap on the infant's head will help decrease these losses. In addition, the use of open bed platforms with radiant warmers as well as phototherapy

**Table 2.1** Factors affecting insensible water loss (IWL) in preterm neonates

---

**Factors that increase IWL**

    Prematurity

    Radiant warmer heat

    Phototherapy

    Skin defects

    Tachypnea

    Non-humidified oxygen

**Factors that decrease IWL**

    Mature skin

    Heat shields

      Plastic wrap blanket

      Rigid plastic body hood

    Topical skin agents

      Paraffin

      Aquaphor

    Covering skin defects

    Humidified oxygen

---

Parish A and Bhatia J. Nutritional considerations in the intensive care unit: neonatal issues. In: SA Shikora, RG Martindale and SD Schwaitzberg, eds. *Nutritional Considerations in the Intensive Care Unit, Science, Rationale and Practice*. Iowa: American Society for Parenteral and Enteral Nutrition, Kendall/Hunt Publishing. Reproduced with permission.

lights increases the IWL by more than 50%. This excessive IWL may be reduced with the use of humidified incubators to care for the infant. The measurement of urine specific gravity has been used to predict urine osmolality. While this is a reliable means of predicting hyperosmolality (urine osmolality of greater than 290 mOsm/kg water with a urine specific gravity 1.012 or greater), it is less helpful in predicting hypo-osmolality (urine osmolality of < 270 mOsm/kg water with a urine specific gravity 1.008 or less). Iso-osmolality is defined by a urine osmolality of 270 to 290 mOsm/kg water with a urine specific gravity 1.008 to 1.012. In addition, glucose and protein in the urine may increase the urine specific gravity, giving a falsely high estimate of urine osmolality. Therefore, when urine specific gravity is evaluated to rule out hyperosmolar urine, glucose and protein in the urine should be measured at the same time. The maximal concentrating capabilities in the neonate are limited compared with those in adults; thus, an infant with a urine osmolality of approximately 700 mOsm/kg water (urine specific gravity of 1.019) may be dehydrated. In practice, this mode of evaluation is not often utilized.

The initial postnatal period is characterized by a relative oliguria for approximately the first 24 hours of life, followed by a diuretic phase that may last 72 hours. These changes are caused by considerable evaporative water loss as well as by continuing diuresis. A brief period of high volume diuresis usually precedes the complete recovery from respiratory distress syndrome. Sodium intake should be restricted in VLBW infants during the period of ECW contraction and generally not added until serum sodium falls below 130 mEq/L. In addition, it should be remembered that despite "no sodium in the fluids," the infant may be inadvertently receiving sodium through the use of saline-containing solutions, calcium gluconate, ampicillin, heparin and sodium bicarbonate. This sodium restriction may assist recovery from respiratory disease and decrease the risk of later chronic lung disease.

## PRACTICAL TIPS for fluid and electrolyte management

1. Initiation of fluid intake at 60 to 80 mL/kg/d on day 1 with 10–20 mL/kg daily increases up to a maximum of 140 mL/kg/d

2 During the first days of life, provide sufficient fluid to result in urine output of 1 to 3 mL/kg/hr, a urine specific gravity of 1.008 to 1.012, evaluating urine for glucose and protein at the same time, and a weight loss of approximately 10 to 15% or less in VLBW infants over the first few days of life

3. If possible, weigh infants twice a day in the first two days of life then daily in order to accurately monitor input and output. The risk–benefit ratio of weighing infants twice a day if "in-bed" scales are not available suggests more risk since infants have to be taken out of their environment to be weighed. Serum sodium can serve as a "proxy" and in the absence of a rapidly rising sodium, fluid adequacy can be ensured

4. Body weight normally reflects changes in TBW, although changes in intravascular volume may be different. Due to "severity of illness" many clinicians use birth weight in order to design fluid therapy until the infant is stable enough to be safely weighed

5. Keep accurate records of fluid intake, output, and weights

6.  Indications of changes of hydration and electrolyte
    status include:
    Clinical status of patient
    Serum concentrations of electrolytes
    Bodyweight
    Fluid balance (water intake and excretion)
    Hct and BUN
    Urine specific gravity
    Urine electrolytes (only if concerned about excessive
       losses)
7.  Na, Cl and K should be supplemented after the first
    3–6 days after birth when contraction occurs (1–2 mEq/
    kg/d). We recommend adding Na when initial level falls
    below 130 mEq/L

## SUGGESTED READING

Bauer K, Bovermann G, Roithmaier A, et al. Body
   composition, nutrition, and fluid balance during the first
   two weeks of life in preterm neonates weighing less than
   1500 grams. *J Pediatr* 1991; **118**:615.

Bell EF, Acarregui MJ, Restricted versus liberal water intake
   for preventing morbidity and mortality in preterm infants
   (Cochrane Review). In: *The Cochrane Library*, Issue 1.
   Chichester, UK: John Wiley; 2004.

Bell EF, Warburton D, Stonestreet BS, et al. High-volume
   fluid intake predisposes premature infants to necrotizing
   enterocolitis. *Lancet* 1979; **2**:90.

Gaylord MS, Wright K, Lorch V, Walker E. Improved fluid management utilizing humidified incubators in extremely low birth weight infants. *J Perinatol* 2001; **21**:438.

Lorenz JM, Kleinman LI, Kotagal UR, et al. Water balance in very low-birth-weight infants: Relationship to water and sodium intake and effect on outcome. *J Pediatr* 1982; **101**:423.

Oh W, Poindexter BB, Perrit MS, et al. Association between fluid intake and weight loss during the first ten days of life and risk of bronchopulmonary dysplasia in extremely low birth weight infants. *J Pediatr* 2005; **147**:786–790.

SINGLETON HOSPITAL
STAFF LIBRARY

# Chapter 3

# Energy

Energy needs are dependent on age, weight, rate of growth, thermal environment, activity, hormonal activity, and organ size and maturation. Because of methodology limitations, resting metabolic rate (RMR) and not true basal metabolic rate is used for VLBW infants (true BMR can only be measured after an overnight fast). The metabolic rate increases during the first weeks of life from an RMR of 40–41 kcal/kg/d during the first week to 62–64 kcal/kg/d by the third week of life. The extra energy expenditure is primarily due to the energy cost of growth related to various synthetic processes. The metabolic rate of the nongrowing infant is approximately 51 kcal/kg/d, which includes 47 kcal/kg/d for basal metabolism and 4 kcal/kg/d for activity.

Exposure of infants to a cold environment significantly increases energy expenditure. For example, infants nursed in an environment just below thermal neutrality increase energy expenditure by 7 to 8 kcal/kg/d. In addition, any stimulation of the infant adds to this energy loss. A daily increase of 10 kcal/kg/d should be allowed to cover incidental cold stress in the preterm infant. Infants who are intrauterine growth restricted, particularly the asymmetrical type, have a higher RMR on a per kilogram body weight basis because of their relatively high proportion of metabolically active mass. Other factors that

**Table 3.1** Estimated energy expenditure in a growing preterm infant

|  | kcal/kg/d |
|---|---|
| Resting energy expenditure | 47 |
| Minimal activity[a] | 4 |
| Occasional cold stress[a] | 10 |
| Fecal loss of energy (10% to 16% of total intake) | 15 |
| Growth[b] (includes dietary-induced thermogenesis) | 45 |
| **Total** | **121** |

[a] As an infant matures, energy expended in activities, such as crying and nursing, increases; at the same time, energy expended as a result of cold stress decreases.

[b] Calculated assuming 3.0 to 4.5 kcal/g weight gain at rate of gain of 10 to 15 g/kg/d.

American Academy of Pediatrics Committee on Nutrition. Nutritional needs of low-birthweight infants. Pediatrics 1985; 75:976. Reproduced with permission.

may increase metabolic rate may include the effects of fever, sepsis, and surgery.

Caloric intake above maintenance is used for growth (Table 3.1). On average each 1-g increment in weight requires 4.5 kcal above maintenance energy. Therefore on enteral nutrition, to attain the equivalent of the third-trimester intrauterine weight gain (15 g/kg/d), a metabolizable energy intake of approximately 70 kcal/kg/d above the 51 kcal/kg/d required for maintenance must be provided, or approximately 120 kcal/kg/d. Increasing metabolizable energy intakes beyond 120 kcal/kg/d with just energy supplementation does not result in proportionate increases in weight gain. However, when energy, protein, fat, and minerals are all increased, weight gain will increase with accretion of protein and fat. Avoiding excessive intakes of carbohydrate energy beyond requirement will also lessen the deposition of fat. The higher the caloric intake, the greater is the amount of energy expended through excretion, dietary-induced thermogenesis, and tissue synthesis. The energy cost of weight gain at 130 kcal/kg/d was reported to be 3.0 kcal/g of weight gain. However, at much higher intakes of energy, 149 kcal/kg/d and 181 kcal/ kg/d, the energy cost of weight gain was estimated to be 4.9 and 5.7 kcal/g of weight gain, respectively.

Infants receiving total parenteral nutrition (TPN) have different energy requirements than the enterally fed infant because there is no fecal loss of nutrients. Preterm infants who are appropriately grown for age are in positive nitrogen balance when receiving 50 nonprotein kilocalories (NPCs)/kg/d along with 2.5 g protein/kg/d. At an NPC intake of greater than 70 kcal/kg/d and a protein intake of 2.7 to 3.5 g/kg/d, preterm infants exhibit nitrogen accretion and growth rates similar to in utero levels. The source of energy for parenteral nutrition in infants is either as glucose or lipid, or a combination of the two. Although both glucose and fat provide equivalent nitrogen-sparing effects in the neonate, studies have demonstrated that a nutrient mixture using intravenous glucose and lipid so-called "balanced TPN" as the nonprotein energy sources is more physiologic than supplying glucose as the only nonprotein energy source. If excess glucose is administered it is converted to fat or triglycerides. Thus a nutrient mixture with both glucose and lipid providing NPCs as well as essential fatty acids is  suggested.

Energy expenditure measurements in critically ill VLBW infants on assisted ventilation are extremely difficult studies to perform using any existing measurement techniques. Leitch and Denne (2000) reviewed 12 studies, with 29 of 75 patients studied in the first 2 to 3 days of life. These studies suggest a mean energy expenditure of approximately 54 kcal/kg. However, technical limitations hampered these investigations, including the inspired oxygen level at which the patients could be studied. Smaller infants had lower energy intakes but also lower energy expenditure of the same magnitude. Since critically ill preterm infants have limited energy stores, it is important to provide adequate energy sources early.

## PRACTICAL TIPS for energy

1. Dextrose calories not to exceed 50% of total calories on TPN
2. Calories from lipids not to exceed 40% of total calories on TPN
3. Calories from protein not to exceed 12% of total calories in TPN
4. Achieving adequate growth with TPN is possible with protein intake approximating 3.0–3.5 g/kg/d; 80–100 kcal/kg/d
5. Excessive energy administration TPN of carbohydrate and lipid can lead to metabolic intolerance including hypertriglyceridemia, acidosis and excessive fat deposition, especially in the liver

6. Infants who are SGA or IUGR and infants developing BPD may need as much as 25–45% more energy: the former due to increased RMR and the latter due to increased expenditure due to work of breathing

## SUGGESTED READING

Bauer, J, Hentschel R, Linderkamp O. Effect of sepsis syndrome on neonatal oxygen consumption and energy expenditure. *Pediatrics* 2002; **110**:e69.

Chessex P, Reichman BL, Verellen GJE, et al. Influence of postnatal age, energy intake, and weight gain on energy metabolism in the very-low-birth weight infant. *J Pediatr* 1981; **99**:761.

Gudinchet F, Schutz Y, Micheli JL. Metabolic cost of growth in very low-birth-weight infants. *Pediatr Res* 1982; **16**:1025.

Heird WC, Hay W, Helms RA, et al. Pediatric parenteral amino acid mixture in low birth weight infants. *Pediatrics* 1988; **81**:41.

Leitch CA, Denne SC. Energy expenditure in the extremely low birth weight infant. *Clin Perinatol* 2000; **27**:181.

Roberts SB, Young VR. Energy costs of fat and protein deposition in the human infant. *Am J Clin Nutr* 1988; **48**:951.

# Chapter 4

# Intravenous carbohydrates

The glucose infusion rate should maintain euglycemia. Glucose intolerance, defined as inability to maintain euglycemia at glucose administration rates < 6 mg/kg/min, is a frequent problem in VLBW infants, and especially in ELBW infants. The plasma glucose concentration should be kept below 130 mg/dL. This hyperglycemia in ELBW infants may also occur in combination with nonoliguric hyperkalemia. As discussed later (Chapter 6), these co-morbidities may be prevented with the early use of TPN.

Endogenous glucose production is elevated in VLBW infants compared with term infants and adults. High glucose production rates are found in VLBW infants who received only glucose compared to those receiving glucose plus amino acids and/or lipids. Clinical experience with hyperglycemia suggests that administration of glucose alone does not always suppress glucose production in VLBW infants. It appears that persistent glucose production is the main cause of hyperglycemia and is fueled by ongoing proteolysis that is not suppressed by physiologic concentrations of insulin. In addition, abnormally low peripheral glucose utilization may also contribute to hyperglycemia. Therefore a 5% glucose concentration instead of the standard 10% concentration of glucose may have to be used in more immature ELBW infants (<750 g).

Glucose intolerance can limit delivery of energy to the infant to a fraction of the resting energy expenditure, resulting in negative energy balance. Several strategies are used to manage this early hyperglycemia in ELBW infants as well as to increase energy intake.

1. Decreasing glucose administration until hyperglycemia resolves (unless the hyperglycemia is so severe that this strategy would require infusion of a hypotonic solution).
2. Administering intravenous amino acids, which decrease serum glucose concentrations in ELBW infants, presumably by enhancing endogenous insulin secretion.
3. Initiation of exogenous insulin therapy at rates to control hyperglycemia (plasma glucose >130 mg/dL at glucose infusion rate (GIR) < 6 mg/kg/min).
4. Using exogenous insulin to increase energy intake.

The first and third strategies prevent adequate early nutrition and the safety of the last has been questioned in this population because of the possible development of lactic acidemia.

Several studies have shown that insulin, used as a nutritional adjuvant, i.e. to increase energy intake, successfully lowers glucose concentrations and increases weight gain in preterm infants without significant risk of hypoglycemia. This weight gain was achieved by lipogenesis, conversion of glucose to lipid, as there was no difference in head circumference vs. control infants. This is an inefficient metabolic process and may cause respiratory problems via increased $CO_2$ production when lipogenesis occurs. However, little is known about its effects on the body composition and counter-regulatory hormone concentrations. A recent study examined the effect of insulin using a hyperinsulinemic–euglycemic clamp in ELBW infants receiving only glucose. These infants were normoglycemic prior to the initiation of insulin. The infants demonstrated a significant elevation in plasma lactate concentrations and the development of significant metabolic acidosis. Additionally the infusion of insulin to these ELBW infants did not alter protein dynamics, as, while protein breakdown was decreased, protein synthesis was also diminished to the same degree. There are growing concerns that relatively high energy intakes administered to ELBW infants may result in excess accretion of adipose tissues and could have significant adverse long-term health consequences.

In our experience, the administration of amino acids early after birth prevents hyperglycemia in the majority of ELBW infants. Stimulation of endogenous insulin secretion and increased insulin activity by specific parenteral amino acids such as arginine and leucine may explain how early amino acid therapy prevents hyperglycemia.

This improved tolerance allows for safely providing appropriate energy for growth while avoiding lactic acidemia associated with insulin infusion in euglycemic infants. Excessive glucose intake above 18 g/kg/d and inducing lipogenesis may adversely affect respiratory gas exchange through increasing $VCO_2$. Oxidation of carbohydrates produces more carbon dioxide then does oxidation of lipids.

Normally, this $CO_2$ is eliminated by increasing respiratory rate. However, in compromised preterm infants, the ability to "blow-off" $CO_2$ may be limited.

## PRACTICAL TIPS for carbohydrates

1. Carbohydrates should provide 50% of total calories
2. Glucose infusion rate will depend on the volume of fluid and the percent dextrose chosen. As the amount of fluid is changed, the amount of glucose infused will change
3. A steady infusion of 6–8 mg/kg/minute of glucose should be provided parenterally
4. Glucose infusion rate (GIR): % glucose × total mL × 1000 mg ÷ 1440 (minutes per day) ÷ weight in kg = mg/kg/minute. Example 1.5 kg infant receives 125 mL/kg D10W (10% dextrose) × 187.5 mL (total fluid) = 18.75 × 1000 = 18750; 18750 ÷ 1440 (minutes in day) = 13.0 mg/day 13.0 ÷ 1.5 = 8.7 mg/kg/minute
5. Use regular insulin for hyperglycemia (serum glucose > 150–200) at GIR <6 mg/kg/minute
6. Insulin bolus 0.1 units per dose
7. Increases in 0.1 units
8. Adjust insulin to maintain serum glucose ≤ 150
9. Administer every 4–6 hours or utilize an insulin drip

ALTERNATIVE

10. Constant infusion 0.1 unit for each 20 g of glucose. This is the best strategy for ELBW infants (<1000 g)

MONITORING

11. Frequently, every 15 minutes × 4 after a bolus, then every 2 hours while receiving insulin
12. Prophylactic infusion of insulin to increase glucose utilization in euglycemic infant does not increase protein balance. It decreases proteolysis and protein synthesis by approximately 20%
13. Excessive glucose intake $\geq$ 18 g/kg/per day or $\geq$ 13 mg/kg/min, 60 kcal/kg/per day as glucose increases $VCO_2$ twice as much as $VO_2$ and may adversely affect respiratory gas exchange. Excessive energy as glucose induces lipogenesis, which is inefficient and increases energy expenditure
14. Glucose intake levels at or below energy expenditure have no effect on respiratory gas exchange

## SUGGESTED READING

Adamkin DH. Pragmatic approach to in-hospital nutrition in high risk neonates. *J Perinatol* 2005; **25**(suppl):S7–S11.

Bhatia J, Gates A. *Neonatal Nutritional Handbook* 6th ed. 2006.

Binder ND, Raschko PK, Benda GI, et al. Insulin infusion with parenteral nutrition in extremely-low-birth-weight infants with hyperglycemia. *J Pediatr* 1989; **144**:273.

Collins JW Jr, Hoppe M, Brown K. A controlled trial of insulin infusion and parenteral nutrition in extremely-low-birth-weight infants with glucose intolerance. *J Pediatr* 1991; **118**:921.

Forsyth JS, Crighton A. Low birthweight infants and total parenteral nutrition immediately after birth. I. Energy expenditure and respiratory quotient of ventilated and non-ventilated infants. *Arch Dis Child Fetal Neonatal Ed* 1995; **73**:F4–7.

Michelli JL, Schutz Y, Jund S, Calame A. Early postnatal amino acid administration in ELBW preterm infants. *Seminars in Neonatal Nutrition and Metabolism*. 1994; **2**:1.

Poindexter BB, Karn CA, Ahlrichs JA, et al. Amino acids suppress proteolysis independent of insulin throughout the neonatal period. *Am J Physiol* 1997; **272**:R592.

Poindexter, BB, Karn, CA, Denne, SC. Exogenous insulin reduces proteolysis and protein synthesis in extremely low birth weight infants. *J Pediatr* 1998; **132**:948–953.

Stefano JL, Norman ME, Morales MC, et al. Decreased erythrocyte Na-K+-ATPase activity associated with cellular potassium loss in extremely-low-birth-weight infants with nonoliguric hyperkalemia. *J Pediatr* 1993; **122**:276.

# Chapter 5

# Intravenous lipids

The use of intravenous lipids is essential to a complete TPN regimen. Lipids serve as a source of linoleic acid to prevent or treat essential fatty acid deficiency (EFAD), and as an energy source. Larger quantities serve as a partial replacement for glucose as a major source of calories (balanced TPN).

The VLBW infant is especially susceptible to the development of EFAD because tissue stores of linoleic acid are small and requirements for essential fatty acids are large secondary to rapid growth. The human fetus depends entirely on placental transfer of essential fatty acids. A VLBW infant with limited nonprotein energy reserve must mobilize fatty acids for energy when receiving intravenous nutrition devoid of lipid. Our own studies in these infants confirm other studies that show that biochemical evidence of EFAD can develop in the VLBW infant during the first week of life on lipid-free regimens.

Standard 20% emulsions contain a lower phospholipids emulsifier/triglycerides ratio than standard 10% lipid emulsions and should preferably be used for TPN. Clearance of lipid emulsions from the blood depends on the activity of lipoprotein lipase. Post-heparin lipoprotein lipase activity can be increased by relatively high doses of heparin; heparin does not improve utilization of intravenous lipids. Therefore the increase in lipase activity by heparin lends to an increase in FFAs which may exceed the infants ability to clear the products of lipolysis. The premature infant can clear 0.15 to 0.2 g/kg/hr of lipids. However, small for gestational age infants and infants with sepsis may not be able to clear standard doses of intravenous lipids and demonstrate hypertriglyceridemia.

The "routine" use of intravenous lipid emulsions has not been universally accepted in critically ill, ventilated VLBW infants because of potential complications. These complications to the ventilated VLBW infant include adverse effects on gas exchange and displacement of bilirubin from albumin. Both Brans et al. (1986) and Adamkin (1986) found no difference in oxygenation between infants randomly assigned to various lipid doses (including controls without lipids) when using lower rates and longer infusion times of intravenous lipids. The displacement of bilirubin from binding sites on serum albumin may occur even with adequate metabolism of infused lipid. In vitro, displacement of ALB-bound bilirubin by FFA depends on the relative concentrations of all three compounds. An in vivo study has shown no free bilirubin generated if the molar FFA/ALB ratio is less than 6. Our data with lipid initiation at 0.5 g/kg/d of lipid in VLBW infants on assisted ventilation with respiratory distress syndrome showed a mean FFA/ALB ratio of less than 1; no individual patient value exceeded a ratio of 3 when daily doses were increased to 2.5 g/kg/d (in increments of 0.5 g/kg/d) over an 18-hour infusion time. Other investigators found no adverse effect on bilirubin binding when lipid emulsion was infused at a dose of 2 g/kg/d over either 15 or 24 hours. Proper use includes slow infusion rates (≤0.125 g/kg/hr), slow increases in dosage, and avoidance of unduly high doses, e.g. >3.0 g/kg/d. Gilbertson et al. (1991) demonstrated that slow administration of intravenous lipids beginning on day 1 at a dose of 1.0 g/kg/d and increasing in stepwise fashion to 3.0 g/kg/d by day 4 is well tolerated without noticeable adverse effects. Also, there were no differences in plasma levels of triglycerides and non-esterified fatty acids compared with infants who did not receive intravenous lipids. Nonetheless, serum triglycerides should be monitored with every increase of lipid intake, at maximum dose and periodically thereafter. Serum triglycerides below 200 mg/dL should be the goal.

Concerns have been raised regarding the possible adverse effects of IVL on pulmonary function, especially in premature neonates and those with acute lung injury. A potential hazard of hyperlipidemia resulting from failure to clear infused lipid is the adverse effect on gas exchange in the lungs. This was demonstrated in adult volunteers after a large dose of soybean emulsion. Preterm neonates randomized to different lipid infusion rates did not demonstrate any effect on alveolar–arterial oxygen gradient or arterial blood pH. Similarly, we found no difference in oxygenation in preterm infants randomly assigned to modest doses of lipids (0.6 to 1.4 g/kg/d) over the first week of life.

For the late-preterm infant who has increased pulmonary vascular resistance (PVR) and/or respiratory disease, it

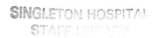
SINGLETON HOSPITAL
STAFF LIBRARY

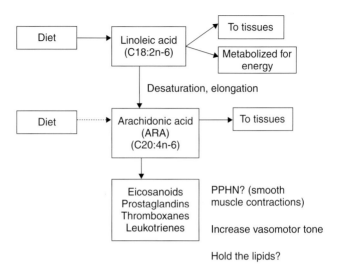

**Figure 5.1** Metabolic derivatives of linoleic acid and ARA. Adamkin DH. *Clin Perinatol* Dec 2006. Reproduced with permission from Elsevier.

appears a more prudent approach with IVL should be taken. Significant concerns have been raised because of the high polyunsaturated fatty acid content (PUFA) of lipid emulsions as the omega–6 (linoleic acid, 18:2n – 6). It is converted to arachidonic acid whose pathways may lead to the synthesis of prostaglandins, leukotrienes and thromboxanes (Fig. 5.1). It is believed the IVL infusion may enhance the activity of these vasoactive eicosanoids, leading to changes in vasomotor tone with resultant hypoxemia, i.e. exacerbate pulmonary hypertension. In addition, the production of hydroperoxides in the lipid emulsion also might contribute to untoward effects by increasing prostaglandin levels.

There is no evidence of adverse effects of lipid emulsions in infants with severe acute respiratory failure with or without pulmonary hypertension (PPHN).

Low plasma carnitine levels are commonly observed in infants and adults receiving carnitine-free TPN, which may inhibit fatty acid oxidation. However, most trials of carnitine supplementation have shown little, if any, effect on fatty acid oxidation. However, carnitine supplementation after about two weeks of carnitine-free TPN is suggested.

## PRACTICAL TIPS for intravenous lipids

1. Use of 20% lipid emulsion to decrease risk of hypertriglyceridemia, hypercholesterolemia and hyperphospholipidemia
2. Fat is a concentrated energy source providing 2 kcal/mL in a 20% lipid emulsion
3. Initiate lipids the day following birth after the initiation of the amino acid stock solution at starting dose of 0.5 or 1.0 g/kg/d or with first TPN if lipids are available via pharmacy. This dose will prevent EFAD
4. Plasma triglycerides are monitored after each increase in dose and levels are maintained less than 200 mg/dL
5. Maximum lipid dosage is usually 3 g/kg/d
6. Lipid infusion hourly rate correlates best with plasma lipid concentrations. Hourly infusion should not exceed 0.15–0.20 g/kg/hr

7. The use of carnitine to increase oxidation of fat is recommended only for low birthweight infants who require (over 2–4 weeks of) parenteral nutrition; I.V. carnitine dosage is 8–10 mg/kg

## SUGGESTED READING

Adamkin DH. Use of intravenous fat emulsions, Part 1. *Perinatol Neonatol* 1986; May/June: 65–190.

Adamkin DH. Feeding the preterm infant. In: J Bhatia, ed. *Perinatal Nutrition: Optimizing Infant Health and Development.* New York: Marcel Dekker; 2004: 1.

Brans YW, Dutton EB, Drew DS, et al. Fat emulsion tolerance in very low birthweight neonates: Effect on diffusion of oxygen in the lungs and on blood pH. *Pediatrics* 1986; **78**:79.

Gilbertson N, Kovar IZ, Cox DJ, et al. Introduction of intravenous lipid administration on the first day of life in the very low birth weight neonate. *J Pediatr* 1991; **119**:615.

Helbock HJ, Motchnik PA, Ames BN. Toxic hydroperoxide in intravenous lipid emulsions used in preterm infants. *Pediatrics* 1993; **91**:83.

Helms RA, Whitington PF, Mauer EC.et al. Enhanced lipid utilization in infants receiving oral L-carnitine during long-term parenteral nutrition. *J Pediatr* 1986; **109**:984–988.

Hunt CE, Pachman LM, Hageman Jr, et al. Liposyn infusion increases prostaglandin concentrations. *Pediatr Pulmonol* 1986; **2**:154.

Lavoic JC, Chessex P. The increase in vasomotor tone induced by a parenteral lipid emulsion is linked to an inhibition of prostacyclin production. *Free Radio Biol Med* 1994; **16**:795.

Spear ML Stahl GE, Hamosh M, et al. Effect of heparin dose and infusion rate on lipid clearance in very low-birth-weight infants. *J Pediatr* 1988; **112**:94–98.

Starinsky R, Shafrir E. Displacement of albumin-bound bilirubin by free fatty acids: Implications for neonatal hyperbilirubinemia. *Clin Chim Acta* 1970; **29**:311.

# Chapter 6

# Early total parenteral nutrition (TPN)

Aggressive nutritional therapy theoretically allows the transition from fetal to extrauterine life to occur with minimal, if any, interruption of growth and development (see Fig. 6.1). However, this aggressive nutritional therapy requires that the transfer of nutrients to the fetus/infant not be interrupted. When birth occurs, particularly in ELBW infants, there is some temporary interruption of the transfer of nutrients. Reduction of this interruption to a reasonable minimum is the first goal of aggressive nutrition. Until recently, the initiation of TPN had been delayed by a number of days. Reasons for such a delay have not been clear but probably have been related to clinicians' perception that the VLBW infant was unable to catabolize amino acids and general concerns about metabolic "tolerance" in the first days after birth for critically ill infants.

Identifying strategies that provide the best foundation to improve growth and developmental outcomes and to reduce complications and morbidities begins with early administration of amino acids. The administration of amino acids from the first postnatal hours to avoid a period of early malnutrition is the first critical strategy to prevent growth failure in ELBW infants and to promote enhanced neurodevelopment (see Fig. 6.2).

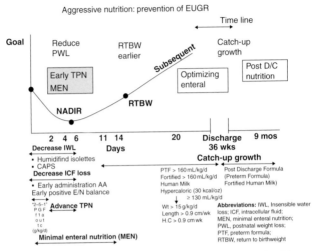

Figure 6.1 Aggressive nutrition: prevention of EUGR. Adamkin DH. Feeding the preterm infant. In: J Bhatia, ed. *Perinatal Nutrition Optimizing Infant Health and Development*. New York, NY: Marcel Dekker; 2004: 165–190. Reproduced with permission.

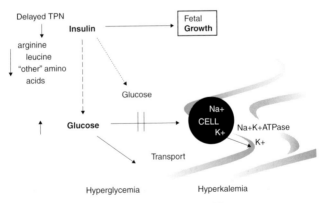

Figure 6.2 Early administration of amino acids.

An understanding of fetal nutrition is helpful in designing postnatal strategies for ELBW infants. At 28 weeks gestation, there is little fetal lipid uptake. Fetal energy metabolism is not dependent on fat until early in the third trimester, and it then increases only gradually toward term. Glucose is delivered to the fetus from the mother at low fetal insulin concentrations, generally at a rate that matches fetal energy expenditure. The human placenta actively transports amino acids to the fetus, and animal studies indicate that fetal amino acid uptake greatly exceeds protein accretion requirements. Approximately 50% of the amino acids taken up by the fetus are oxidized and serve as a significant source of energy. Urea production is a byproduct of amino acid oxidation. Relatively high rates of fetal urea production are seen in human and animal fetuses compared with the term neonate and adult, suggesting that high protein turnover and oxidation rates occur in the fetus. An increase in blood urea nitrogen, which is often observed after the start of TPN, is not an adverse effect or sign of toxicity; rather, it is related to an increase in the intake of amino acids or protein. Several controlled studies have demonstrated the efficacy and safety of amino acids initiated within the first 24 hours after birth. No recognizable metabolic derangements, including hyperammonemia, metabolic acidosis, or abnormal aminograms, were observed. A strong argument for the early aggressive use of amino acids is the prevention of "metabolic shock." Concentrations of some key amino acids begin to decline in the VLBW infant from the time the umbilical cord is cut and placental transfer of nutrients is halted. Such metabolic shock may trigger the starvation response, of which endogenous glucose production is a prominent feature. Irrepressible glucose production may be the cause of the so-called glucose intolerance that often limits the amount of energy that can be administered to the VLBW infant. It is prudent to support the metabolic transition from fetal to extrauterine life rather than to withhold TPN and send the infant into a metabolic emergency. The need for TPN may never be more acute than immediately after birth. Another benefit of this strategy was recognized when investigators observed that glucose tolerance improves substantially in infants receiving early amino acids. This would safely allow the provision of more nonprotein energy while avoiding hyperglycemia.

Early amino acid administration may stimulate insulin secretion, consistent with the concept that forestalling the starvation response improves glucose tolerance. The mechanism may be that without initiation of early parenteral amino acids, plasma concentrations of certain amino acids (e.g. arginine and leucine) decrease. Secretion of insulin depends on the plasma concentrations of these amino acids as well as that of glucose. A shortage of amino acids limits the secretion and activity of insulin. Finally, glucose transport and energy metabolism is adversely affected by a reduction in insulin and insulin-like growth factors. This scenario leads to a down-regulation of glucose transporters at the cellular membrane level, resulting in intracellular energy failure via a decrease in $Na^+,K^+$ ATPase activity. This directly contributes to leakage of intracellular potassium and is associated with nonoliguric hyperkalemia. Early TPN with amino acids minimizes the abrupt postnatal deprivation of amino acid supply and provides the following benefits:

- Prevention of protein catabolism
- Prevention of a decrease in growth-regulating factors such as insulin and down-regulation of glucose transporters
- Prevention of hyperglycemia and nonoliguric hyperkalemia

From a growth standpoint, this strategy should be associated with less extreme postnatal weight loss and an earlier return to birthweight. An earlier return to birthweight means the VLBW infant will be less likely to develop extrauterine growth restriction. The early provision of amino acids leads to improved nitrogen balance and potentially long-term neurodevelopmental outcomes by improving in-hospital growth velocity and providing overall enhanced nutrition for ELBW infants.

## PRACTICAL TIPS for early total parenteral nutrition (TPN)

1. Early TPN amino acids at dosage of 1.5 to 3.0 g/kg/d maybe initiated within hours of birth. A stock solution of 4% amino acids with dextrose 10% concentration can easily provide an amino acid dosage that replaces ongoing losses as part of the initial fluid provided to the VLBW infant. Alternatively, the dose of amino acids can be "piggy-backed" along with the glucose concentration and delivery chosen by the clinician

2. Intakes up to 4.0 g/kg/d for ELBW infants may be appropriate when enteral feedings are extremely delayed or withheld for prolonged periods. This intake of, amino acids should not exceed 12% of total calories

3. An elevated BUN of up to 40 mg/dL has been observed in neonates early in life with and without TPN. After the initial 5–7 days, an elevated BUN >20 mg/dL may represent excessive amino acid delivery, decreased utilization and subsequent oxidation, or it may represent amino acid intolerance. BUN is a good indicator of protein nutritional status in the absence of renal dysfunction; a BUN of <5mg/dL suggests that amino acid (protein) intake is at or below requirements

4. Modification of amino acid intake should not be based on BUN concentration alone. A continuously rising BUN value may indicate a mismatch between production and excretion

## SUGGESTED READING

Adamkin DH. Pragmatic approach to in-hospital nutrition in high-risk neonates. *J Perinatol* 2005; **25**(suppl):S7–S11.

Adamkin DH. Nutrition management of the very low birthweight infant. *NeoReviews* 2006; 7 (12).

Dinerstein A, Neito RM, Solana CL, et al. Early and aggressive nutritional strategy (parenteral and enteral) decreases postnatal growth failure in very low birth weight infants. *J Perinatol* 2006; **26**:436–442.

Ibraham HM, Jeroudi MA, Baier RJ, et al. Aggressive early total parental nutrition inlow-birth-weight infants. *J Perinatol* 2003; **24**:24–32

Kotsopoulos K, Benadiba-Torch A, Cuddy A, et al. Safety and efficacy of early amino acids in preterm < 28 weeks gestation: prospective observational comparison. *J Perinatol* 2006; **26**:749–754.

te Braake FWJ, Van Den Akker CHP, Wattimena DJL, et al. Amino acid administration to premature infants directly after birth. *J Pediatr* 2005; **147**;457–461.

Thureen PJ, Hay WW Jr. Intravenous nutrition and postnatal growth of the micropremie. *Clin Perinatol* 2000; **27**:197–219.

Thureen PJ, Melara D, Fennessey PV, et al. Effect of low versus high intravenous amino acid intake on very low birth weight infants in the early neonatal period. *Pediatr Res* 2003; **53**:24–32.

Ziegler EE, Thureen PJ, Carlson SJ. Aggressive nutrition of the very-low-birth-weight infant. *Clin Perinatol* 2002; **29**:225–244.

# Chapter 7

# Parenteral calcium, phosphorus, magnesium, and vitamin D

Recommendations for mineral and vitamin D intake for preterm infants are based on metabolic studies with the goal being optimizing bone and mineral homeostasis associated with normal serum minerals and vitamin D metabolites and, most important for the VLBW infant, normal bone density.

The molar Ca:P ratio is 1.3 in the whole body and 1.67 in the bone mineral apatite. Ninety-seven percent of whole body calcium and 80% of whole body phosphorus are stored in the apatite together.

Serum calcium exists in three fractions: ionized calcium (~50%), protein-bound calcium (~40%), and a small amount of calcium that is complexed, primarily to citrate and phosphate ions. Serum calcium is maintained at a constant level by the actions of principally parathyroid hormone and calcitonin.

In the presence of low phosphate intake the kidney retains phosphate and it disappears from the urine. Hypercalcemia and hypercalciuria may result from phosphate deficiency. Deficiency of phosphate results in bone demineralization and osteopenia of prematurity. Calcium is actively transported across the placenta in the third trimester of gestation; thus an infant born in the third trimester, especially early in that trimester, is born relatively osteopenic and strategies to maintain calcium homeostasis are of paramount importance.

TPN for VLBW infants typically provides minerals to meet about 60–70% of intrauterine mineral requirements. Early TPN when reaching volumes of 120–130 mL/kg/d contains calcium at 60–90 mg/kg/d, phosphorus at 47–70 mg/kg/d, magnesium at 4.3–7.2 mg/kg/d and vitamin D at 40–160 IU/kg/d (Table 7.1). VLBW infants on TPN for longer duration (> two weeks) should receive an approximate 33% increase in calcium and phosphorus concentration in their infusate.

Several therapies to improve delivery of sufficient amounts of minerals to VLBW infants include using organic salts (calcium gluconate or gluceptate) and organic phosphate salts (sodium glycerophosphate) or glucose monophosphate, decreasing the pH of the solution by using sulfur-containing acidic amino acids (L-cysteine hydrochloride), and mixing phosphate salts before addition of calcium salts. The addition of L-cysteine lowers the pH of the infusate, thus allowing greater calcium solubility.

Use of diuretics, especially long-term, will lead to hypercalciuria and can lead to nephrocalcinosis and increased metabolic bone disease. Aluminum content of infusates such as TPN, albumin etc., has been implicated in metabolic bone disease; however, given the low degree of aluminum contamination in current infusates, aluminum is not an active contributor to altered calcium/phosphorus homeostasis.

**Table 7.1.** Mineral and vitamin D requirements for parenteral nutrition solutions

|         | Ca        | P                                  | Mg       | VIT D                              | CA/P ratio            |
|---------|-----------|------------------------------------|----------|------------------------------------|-----------------------|
|         |           | $(mg\,kg^{-1}\,day^{-1})$          |          | $(IU\,kg^{-1}\,day^{-1})$          | By weight             |
| Term    | 60        | 45                                 | 7        | 40–160                             | 1.3:1–1.7:1           |
|         |           | $(mmol\,kg^{-1}\,day^{-1})$        |          | $(\mu g/day)$                      | Molar                 |
|         | 1.25–1.5  | 1.25–1.5                           | 0.3      | 1.0–4.0                            | 1:1–1.3:1             |
|         |           | $(mg\,kg^{-1}\,day^{-1})$          |          | $(IU\,kg^{-1}\,day^{-1})$          | By weight             |
| Preterm | 60–90     | 47–70                              | 4.3–7.2  | 40–160                             | 1.3:1–1.7:1           |
|         |           | $(mmol\,kg^{-1}\,day^{-1})$        |          | $(\mu g\,day^{-1})$                | Molar                 |
|         | 1.5–2.25  | 1.5–2.25                           | 0.18–0.3 | 1.0–4.0                            | 1:1–1.3:1             |

From Itani O, Tsang R. Disorders of mineral, vitamin D and bone homeostasis. In: P.J. Thureen and W.W. Hay, eds. *Neonatal Nutrition and Metabolism*. Cambridge University Press; 2006. Reproduced with permission.

*Note*: Ca and P concentrations are based on fluid intake of 120–150 mL/kg/day. Precipitation may occur with concentrations above 60 mg/dL of calcium and 45 mg/dL of phosphate.

1.0 mmol of phosphate = 96 mg.

1 mEq of elemental ccalcium = 20 mg.

1 μg of vitamin D = 40 IU.

## PRACTICAL TIPS for parenteral calcium, phosphorus, magnesium and vitamin D

1. I.V. calcium supplement to all infants BW ≤ 1800 grams upon admission until TPN established. Dose of elemental calcium 200 mg/kg/d

2. One mL of calcium gluconate contains 10 mg/mL of elemental calcium or 1000 mg/mL of the calcium salt

3. Ca:P ratio of 1.3 to 1.7:1 by weight and 1:1 molar ratio is associated with stable bone and mineral homeostasis
4. After the third day, check the phosphorus level along with the calcium level in the event of hypocalcemia
5. Check serum magnesium if hypocalcemia does not respond to therapy
6. Check the I.V. site at least once/hour when high concentrations of calcium are utilized in order to minimize the serious complications of I.V. sloughs
7. Alkaline phosphatase (SAP), phosphorus and calcium levels are checked after two weeks of exclusive TPN; the rate-limiting nutrient for the development of metabolic bone disease is phosphorus, not calcium or vitamin D
8. Signs of deficiencies of calcium include neonatal seizures, decreased bone density, rickets, osteopenia, and tetany
9. Signs of deficiencies of phosphorus include seizures, decreased bone density, rickets, bone pain, and decreased cardiac function

## SUGGESTED READING

Eggert LD, Rusho WJ, Mackay MW, et al. Calcium and phosphate compatibility in parenteral nutritional containing TrophAmine. *Am J Hosp Pharm* 1986; **43**:88.

Gates A, Bhatia J. *Neonatal Nutrition Handbook*. 6th ed. 2006.

Greene HL, Hambidge KM, Schanler R, et al. Guidelines for the use of vitamins, trace elements, calcium, magnesium, and phosphorus in infants and children receiving total parenteral nutrition: Report of the Subcommittee on Pediatric Parenteral Nutrient Requirements from the Committee on Clinical Practice Issues of The American Society for Clinical Nutrition. *Am J Clin Nutr* 1988; **48**:1324.

Koo WW, Tsang RC, Streichen JJ et al. Parenteral nutrition for infants: effect of high versus low calcium and phosphorus content. *J Pediatr Gastroenterol Nutr* 1987; **6**:96–104.

Prestridge LL, Schanler RJ, Shulman RJ, Burns PA, Laine LL. Effect of parenteral calcium and phosphorus therapy on mineral retention and bone mineral content in very low birth weight infants. *J Pediatr* 1993; **122**:761–768.

# Chapter 8

# Parenteral vitamins

Multivitamin infusates are the source used for TPN in VLBW infants. Consideration of vitamins adhering to tubing or being photodegraded by light is an issue of importance in VLBW infants. For example, vitamin A is the most vulnerable to degradation by light and therefore the quantity delivered to the patient may be much lower than the intended dose, particularly when slow infusion rates are used in VLBW infants. Similarly, amino acids and lipids have been demonstrated to be affected by light-exposed TPN solutions containing vitamins, especially riboflavin. However, these changes, although implicated in both hepatic dysfunction and bronchopulmonary dysplasia, remain theoretical.

The optimal requirement for vitamins in neonates has not been determined. Additionally there are only a few multivitamin preparations available for VLBW infants. Surprisingly, there has been little new information relating to vitamins in TPN for VLBW infants over the last 20 years. It is recommended to maintain TPN vitamin dosages that have been previously recommended (Tables 8.1 and 8.2) and are essentially based on expert opinion. Vitamins A and E, fat-soluble vitamins, are of particular interest in VLBW infants.

**Table 8.1** Recommended intakes for parenteral supply of lipid-soluble vitamins for infants and children

|  | Infants (dose/kg body weight per day) | Children (dose per day) |
| --- | --- | --- |
| Vitamin A (µg)[a] | 150–300 | 150 |
| Vitamin D (µg) | 0.8 (32 IU) | 10 (400 IU) |
| Vitamin E (mg) | 2.8–3.5 | 7 |
| Viamin K (µg) | 10 recommended, but currently not possible | 200 |

[a] 1 µg RE (retinol equivalent) =1 µg all trans retinol = 3.33 IU vitamin A.
From Koletzko B, Goulet O, Shamir R. ESPGHAN, ESPEN Guidelines on Paediatric Parenteral Nutrition. *JPGN* 2005; 41;suppl 2.

**Table 8.2** Recommended intakes for parenteral supply of water-soluble vitamins for infants and children

|  | Infants (dose/kg body weight per day) | Children (dose per day) |
| --- | --- | --- |
| Ascorbic acid (mg) | 15–25 | 80 |
| Thiamine (mg) | 0.35–0.50 | 1.2 |
| Riboflavin (mg) | 0.15–0.2 | 1.4 |
| Pyridoxine (mg) | 0.15–0.2 | 1.0 |
| Niacin (mg) | 4.0–6.8 | 17 |
| B12 (µg) | 0.3 | 1 |
| Pantothenic acid (mg) | 1.0–2.0 | 5 |
| Biotin (µg) | 5.0–8.0 | 20 |
| Folic acid (µg) | 56 | 140 |

From Koletzko B, Goulet O, Shamir R. ESPGHAN, ESPEN Guidelines on Paediatric Parenteral Nutrition. *JPGN* 2005; 41;suppl 2. Reproduced with permission.

## Vitamin A

Vitamin A has an essential role in normal differentiation and maintenance of epithelial cells. Prophylactic supplementation with the vitamin was reported to protect against bronchopulmonary dysplasia and to reduce the requirement of oxygen in preterm infants. Serum concentrations below 200 µg/L have been considered to indicate deficiency and levels below 100 µg/L indicate severe deficiency and depleted liver stores in preterm infants.

In infants, an intravenous vitamin A supply of about 920 IU/kg/d together with the water-soluble mixture or 230–500 IU/kg/d with the lipid emulsion are often used. The amount received by the patient after consideration of the losses to light or tube adhesion may be estimated at 300 to 400 IU/kg/d for both options.

For VLBW infants a Cochrane review found an association between vitamin A supply and reduction in death or oxygen requirement at one month of age and of oxygen requirement of survivors at 36 weeks post-menstrual age, with the latter outcome confined to ELBW infants. The NICHD trial included 12 weekly intramuscular injections with 5000 IU of vitamin A to reduce the incidence of BPD. The number to treat is estimated at 13 infants to prevent one infant from developing BPD.

## Vitamin E

Vitamin E is a lipid-soluble antioxidant, protecting cell membrane polyunsaturated fatty acids from free radical oxidative damage. In VLBW infants vitamin E supplementation leading to serum levels >3.5 mg/dL increased the risk of sepsis, but reduced the risk of severe retinopathy of prematurity and intracranial hemorrhage. Evidence does not support the routine application of vitamin E intravenously at high doses to try and achieve serum tocophenol levels >3.5 mg/dL. Safe blood levels for these infants are 1–2 mg/dL.

---

### PRACTICAL TIPS for parenteral vitamins

1. Clinical signs of vitamin deficiencies
   Vitamin D: decreased bone density, osteopenia, rickets
   Vitamin E: mild hemolytic anemia, usually manifesting itself by 4–6 weeks of life, mild edema, thrombosis (this rarely occurs as the LCFUFA to vitamin E ratio in current enteral formulations is adequate)
   Vitamin K: increased prothrombin time, bleeding (petechiae, purpura, ecchymoses, intracranial)
   Folate: megaloblastic anemia, glossitis, diarrhea, irritability
   Thiamin: hyporeflexia, muscle weakness, tachycardia, edema, irritability, Wernicke's encephalopathy
   Biotin: dermatitis, alopecia, irritability, lethargy
2. Vitamin A delivery is improved by the infusion of retinyl pulmitate with lipids, but light-protecting tubing provides only a marginal benefit. However, infusing vitamins with lipids has been demonstrated to result in the production of lipid peroxides. The data to recommend routine addition of vitamins in lipid emusions are inconclusive

3. The administration of multivitamins with the intravenous lipid emulsion provides a practical way to reduce peroxidation of the lipid while limiting vitamin loss

## SUGGESTED READING

Bhatia J, Gates A. *Neonatal Nutrition Handbook*. 6th ed. 2006.

Brion L, Bell E, Raghuveer T. Vitamin E supplementation for prevention of morbidity and mortality in preterm infants. *Cochrane Database Syst Rev* 2003; **4**:CD003665.

Greene HL, Hambidge KM, Schanler R, et al. Guidelines for the use of vitamins, trace elements, calcium, magnesium, and phosphorus in infants and children receiving total parenteral nutrition: Report of the Subcommittee on Pediatric Parenteral Nutrient Requirements from the Committee on Clinical Practice Issues of The American Society for Clinical Nutrition. *Am J Clin Nutr* 1988; **48**:1324.

Koletzko B, Goulet O, Shamir R. ESPGHAN, ESPEN Guidelines on Paediatric Parenteral Nutrition. *JPGN* 2005; 41;suppl 5.

Silvers KM, Sluis KB, Darlow BA, et al. Limiting light-induced lipid peroxidation and vitamin loss in infant parenteral nutrition by adding multivitamin preparations to Intralipid. *Acta Pediatr* 2001; **90**:242–247.

Silvers KM, Darlow BA, Winterbourne CC. Lipid peroxide and hydrogen peroxide formation in parenteral nutrition solutions containing multivitamins. *JPEN J Parenter Enteral Nutr* 2001; **25**:14–17.

# Chapter 9

# Trace elements and iron

Trace elements – chromium, copper, iodine, manganese, molybdenum, selenium, and zinc – are essential micronutrients involved in metabolism in VLBW infants. VLBW infants are at risk for trace element deficiencies because premature birth does not allow adequate transplacental stores and secondly there are the increased demands of rapid growth. TPN trace elements are calculated to prevent the development of deficiency syndromes and to match in-utero accretion rates. The requirements for selenium and zinc in VLBW infants are more controversial (Table 9.1).

## Selenium

Selenium (Se) is an antioxidant as an essential component of active glutathione peroxidase, an enzyme that may protect against oxidative tissue damage. Low Se status has been documented in preterm infants and has been implicated in oxidative diseases such as BPD and/or ROP. It appears that VLBW infants might require twice the amount currently recommended of 1–3 µg/kg/d.

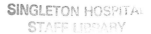
SINGLETON HOSPITAL
STAFF LIBRARY

**Table 9.1** Recommended mineral intakes for very low birthweight infants

| | | ELBW and VLBW | | |
|---|---|---|---|---|
| | | Day 0<br>per kg/d | Transition<br>per kg/d | Growing<br>per kg/d |
| Sodium (mg) | Parenteral | 0–23 | 46–115 | 69–115 (161[a]) |
| | Enteral | 0–23 | 46–115 | 69–115 (161[a]) |
| Potassium (mg) | Parenteral | 0 | 0–78 | 78–117 |
| | Enteral | 0 | 0–78 | 78–117 |
| Chloride (mg) | Parenteral | 0–35.5 | 71–178 | 107–249 |
| | Enteral | 0–35.5 | 71–178 | 107–249 |
| Calcium (mg) | Parenteral | 20–60 | 60 | 60–80 |
| | Enteral | 33–100 | 100 | 100–220 |
| Phosphorus (mg) | Parenteral | 0 | 45–60 | 45–60 |
| | Enteral | 20–60 | 60–140 | 60–140 |
| Magnesium (mg) | Parenteral | 0 | 4.3–7.2 | 4.3–7.2 |
| | Enteral | 2.5–8.0 | 7.9–15.0 | 7.9–15.0 |
| Iron (mg) | Parenteral | 0 | 0 | 0.1–0.2 |
| | Enteral | 0 | 0 | 2.0–4.0 |
| Zinc (µg) | Parenteral | 0–150 | 150 | 400 |
| | Enteral | 0–1000 | 400–1200 | 1000–3000 |
| Copper (µg) | Parenteral | 0 | ≤20 | 20 |
| | Enteral | 0 | ≤150 | 120–150 |
| Selenium (µg) | Parenteral | 0 | ≤1.3 | 1.5–4.5 |
| | Enteral | 0 | ≤1.3 | 1.3–4.5 |

Day 0 = day of birth.

Transition: the period of physiologic and metabolic instability following birth which may last as long as 7 days.

[a] May need up to 160 mg/kg/day for late hyponatremia

Adapted from: Tsang RC, Uauy R, Koletzko B, Zlotkin SH. *Nutrition of the Preterm Infant. Scientific Basis and Practical Guidelines.* 2nd ed. Cincinnati, OH; Digital Educational Publishing; 2005: 415–416. With permission.

## Zinc

Zinc (Zn) is involved in metabolism of energy, the macronutrients, and nucleic acids. It is an essential element for tissue accretion. VLBW infants need more Zn than term infants, because of rapid growth. To match in-utero accretion, 450–500 µg/kg/d is needed. The standard trace element products do not meet this requirement. Therefore, the VLBW infant, and those infants with high zinc losses such as from diarrhea, stomal losses or severe skin disease, need additional zinc sulfate, added to TPN. VLBW infants require an intake of 250 µg/kg/d and therefore Zn is the only trace element that should be added to short-term TPN.

## Iron

Iron is not routinely provided in TPN for VLBW infants. Two major concerns with iron administration with TPN are iron overload and immune function impairment, thereby increasing risk of infection by iron-requiring pathogens. Additionally in the VLBW infant iron has the ability to generate free oxygen radicals. The rich content of double bonds of the lipid emulsion used in TPN may serve as a substrate for iron induced peroxidation in VLBW infants and might increase the risk of BPD.

There is controversy on recommendations as to the need for routine iron supplementation for VLBW infants on TPN. VLBW infants have low iron stores and rapid growth. Although iron stores at birth should be adequate to supply red blood cell production for 3–5 months, iron deficiency has been shown to develop much sooner. While recommendations do exist for iron supplementation to VLBW infants on TPN, we believe a more cautious approach as recommended by Georgieff (2006) is more prudent. Iron delivery should be delayed in VLBW infants receiving initial TPN. For prolonged TPN (>3 weeks) parenteral iron can be provided at 100–200 µg/kg/d.

---

### PRACTICAL TIPS for trace minerals

1. Zinc deficiency is associated with acrodermatitis enteropathical failure to thrive, hypoproteinemia with general edema and increased susceptibility to infection
2. Clinical signs of selenium deficiency include poor growth and cardiomyopathy
3. Clinical signs of iron deficiency include hypochromic microcytic anemia, pallor and tachycardia

---

### SUGGESTED READING

Georgieff MK. Iron. In: PJ Thureen and WW Hay, eds. *Neonatal Nutrition and Metabolism*. Cambridge University Press; 2006.

Greene HL, Hambidge KM, Schanler R, et al. Guidelines for the use of vitamins, trace elements, calcium, magnesium, and phosphorus in infants and children receiving total parenteral nutrition: Report of the Subcommittee on Pediatric Parenteral Nutrient Requirements from the Committee on Clinical Practice Issues of The American Society for Clinical Nutrition. *Am J Clin Nutr* 1988; **48**:1324.

Papageorgiou T, Zacharoulis D, Xenos D, et al. Determination of trace elements (Cu, Zn, Mn, Pb) and magnesium by atomical absorption in patients receiving total parenteral nutrition. *Nutrition* 2002; **18**:32–34.

Schanler RJ, Shulman RJ, Prestidge LL. Pareneral nutrient needs of very low birth weight infants. *J Pediatr* 1994; **125**:961–968.

# Chapter 10

# Parenteral nutrition guide

Early TPN should promote the overall nutritional health of the VLBW infant as evidenced by enhanced neurodevelopmental outcomes and growth at 18–22 months. In addition, males receiving early aggressive TPN showed improved head circumference growth at 18 months of age.

Early TPN affects growth by decreasing the magnitude of the nadir of postnatal weight loss and supporting an earlier return to birthweight. This early growth advantage contributes to less postnatal growth failure and extrauterine growth restriction.

Table 10.1 is the overall guide to providing TPN to VLBW infants. It is followed by Table 10.2, which assesses safety and tolerance to TPN with appropriate laboratory tests. Table 10.3 details the weaning TPN process as enteral nutrition is initiated and advanced, enabling the balance of fat, carbohydrates and protein.

**Table 10.1** Parenteral nutrition guide

| Nutrient | Standard | Advance by | Acceptable labs | Notes |
|---|---|---|---|---|
| Fluid | DOL1–3: 80–100 mL/kg<br>DOL4: 100–120 mL/kg<br>DOL5: 130–150 mL/kg | Increase by 10–20 mL/kg/d | Na 130–145 mEq/L<br>K 3.5–5.5 mEq/L | Adjust fluid based on I & Os and electrolytes and weight |
| Dextrose | Peripheral: D10–12.5%<br>Central: D10–15% | Adjust as fluid is changed keeping glucose delivery at 6–8 mg/kg/min | Glucose 45–130 mg/dL | Dextrose calories not to exceed 50% of total calories |
| Lipids | 3 g/kg/d | Begin with 1 g/kg/d and increase by 1 g/kg/d until goal is met | Triglycerides ≤ 200 mg/dL | Calories from fat not to exceed 40% of total calories |
| Protein | 3 g/kg/d | Begin with 2.0–3 g/kg and increase by 1 g/kg/d until goal is met | BUN* 6–40 mg/dL, individualized approach creatinine 0.8–1.2 mg/dL | Calories from protein not to exceed 12% of total calories |
| Cysteine | 40 mg/g of amino acid | | | Not to exceed 100 mg/kg/d |
| Carnitine | 8 mg/kg <1250 g begin on DOL14 >1250 g begin on DOL30 | | | Carnitine is a cofactor required for the oxidation of fatty acids |
| Sodium | 3 mEq/kg | Adjusts per labs and fluid status | Na 130–145 mg/dL | No sodium until Na level is <130 mg/dL |

| | Dose | Adjustment | Lab range | Notes |
|---|---|---|---|---|
| Potassium | 2 mEq/kg | Adjust per labs and fluid status | K 3.5–5.5 mEq/L | Watch for increase levels in the first few days of life |
| Magnesium | 0.25mEq/dL | Adjust per labs | Mg 1.7–2.1 mg/dL | Maintain a 2:1 ratio with $PO_4$ |
| Calcium | 1–3 mEq/kg | Adjust per solubility and labs | Ca 7.6–10.4 mg/dL ionized Ca | Maintain a 2:1 Ca to $PO_4$ ratio |
| Phosphorus | 0.5–1.5 mEq/kg | Adjust per solubility and labs | $PO_4$ 5–7mg/dL | Chloride can be used to adjust acetate |
| Chloride | 1–2 mEq/kg | Adjust per labs | Cl 95–110 mEq/L | |
| Acetate | 1 mEq/kg | Adjust per labs | $CO_2$ 18–24 mEq/L | Acetate can only be manipulated by decreasing/ increasing chloride |
| Pediatric MVI | 1 mL/kg/d | | | Given to all infants when TPN begins |
| Iron | 200 µg/kg | | | Begin if EPOGEN used or prolongs TPN (>3 wks) |
| Zinc | 200 µg/kg | | | Added to infants weighing <3 kg |
| Iodine | | | | Only given to infants receiving TPN for >4 weeks (1 µg/kg/d) |

**Table 10.1** (*cont.*)

| Nutrient | Standard | Advance by | Acceptable labs | Notes |
|---|---|---|---|---|
| Copper** | 30 µg/kg | | | Added to infants weighing <3 kg |
| Manganese** | 6 µg/kg | | | Added to all TPN |
| Chromium | 0.2 µg/kg | | | Added to all TPN |
| Selenium | 2 µg/kg | | | Added to all TPN |
| Trace pack | 0.2 mL/kg | | | Added to all TPN |
| Heparin | 0.5–0.7 units/mL | | | Maximum 1 unit/mL (100 units/kg) |
| Osmolarity | | | | Not to exceed 1200 mOsm/L in a peripheral line. Adjust protein or sodium if osmolarity is too high |

Adapted and modified from Bhatia I, Gates A. *Neonatal Nutrition Handbook*. 6th ed. 2006.

* BUN: an elevated BUN may represent appropriate amino acid delivery, utilization and subsequent oxidation, or it may represent amino acid intolerance. Modification of amino acid intake should not be based on BUN concentrations alone. A continually rising BUN value may indicate a mismatch between production and excretion.

** Remove if evidence of TPN-associated cholestasis, D Bili > 2.2 mg/dL. Add back weekly if on long-term exclusive TPN.

## Table 10.2  Normal lab values for neonates

| Lab | Normal value |
| --- | --- |
| Sodium, mEq/L | 135–145 |
| Potassium, mEq/L | 3.9–5.9 |
| BUN, mg/dL | 6–40 |
| Creatinine, mg/dL | 0.3–1.2 (can be higher in very sm. Preemies) |
| Chloride, mEq/dL | 95–110 |
| $CO_2$, mEq/dL | 18–24 |
| Glucose, mg/dL | 45–135 |
| Triglyceride, mg/dL | <200 |
| B12, ng/dL (1,25 di-hydroxy) | 12–60 |
| Magnesium, mg/dL | 1.7–2.1 |
| Phosphorus, mg/dL | 5.6–8.5 |
| GGT, U/L | <200 |
| Ionized Calcium, mg/dL | 3.5–5 |
| Calcium, mg/dL | |
| <10 day | 7.5–11.5 |
| 10 days–2 years | 9–10.6 |
| Alkaline phosphotase, U/dL | <300 |
| T. protein, g/dL | 4.2–7.6 |
| Total bilirubin, mg/dL | 1–12 |
| Direct bilirubin, mg/dL | <2.0 |
| AST, MU/dL | 15–60 |
| ALT, MU/mL | 10–70 |
| Hemoglobin, g/dL | 11–17 |
| Hematocrit | 35–49% |
| Reticulocytes | 0–5% |
| Platelets, per μl | 350,000 |

**Table 10.3** Weaning parenteral nutrition enteral feeding volume (preterm formula)

| TPN macronutrients | Goal TPN (NPO) | 20 mL/kg | 40 mL/kg | 60 mL/kg | 80 mL/kg | 100 mL/kg |
|---|---|---|---|---|---|---|
| Amino acids | 3–3.5 | 3–3.5 | 2.5–3 | 2–2.5 | 2 | 0 |
| Lipids (g/kg) | 3–3.5 | 3–3.5 | 2–2.5 | 1.5–2 | 1–1.5 | 0 |
| Glucose delivery (mg/kg/minute) | 6–8 | 6–8 | 6–8 | 6–8 | 6–8 | 6–8[a] |

[a] Supplemental IVF to maintain hydration as enteral feedings advance.

Adapted and modified from Bhatia J, Gates A. *Neonatal Nutrition Handbook*. 6th ed. 2006.

# Chapter 11

# Parenteral nutrition-associated cholestasis in VLBW infants

## Introduction

Neonatal cholestasis is frequently encountered in infants hospitalized for prematurity, gastrointestinal malformations (such as gastroschisis, omphalocele, short gut syndrome, biliary atresia, Alagille syndrome), infection, hemolytic disorders, endocrinopathies (such as hypothyroidism and hypopituitarism), and metabolic abnormalities (such as alpha-1-antitrypsin deficiency, galactosemia). It is common among preterm infants because of immature hepatobiliary function, associated infections, and exposure to hepatotoxic agents such as parenteral alimentation fluids (TPN). Cholestasis is defined as conjugated hyperbilirubinemia (serum conjugated bilirubin concentration greater than 2 mg/dL) because of diminished bile flow and/or excretion of conjugated bilirubin from the hepatocytes into the duodenum. The conjugated fraction of serum bilirubin is normally no greater than 15% of the total serum bilirubin concentration. The incidence of neonatal cholestasis is approximately 1:2500 live births. Once cholestatic liver disease is identified, prompt diagnosis and treatment are necessary.

Cholestasis is a common complication of long-term parenteral nutrition, especially in VLBW infants. If TPN is administered long-term, management should be focused on preventing occurrence of parenteral nutrition-associated cholestasis (PNAC). In this chapter, causes and strategies for reversal and/or prevention of total parenteral nutrition-associated cholestasis (TPNAC) will be discussed.

## Potential causes of TPNAC

TPNAC is the leading cause of neonatal cholestasis and the primary indication for combined liver and intestinal transplantation in children. Within 2 weeks of TPN, biochemical changes in several liver enzymes indicative of hepatic dysfunction appear. Serial measurement of the serum concentration of conjugated bilirubin is necessary to monitor the progression of cholestasis. Alkaline phosphatase and γ-glutamyl transpeptidase (GGT) are sensitive markers for liver disease but lack specificity because concentrations may be elevated in other diseases as well (e.g. osteopenia of prematurity and hepatitis). Elevations of aspartate aminotransferase (AST) and alanine aminotransferase (ALT) reflect hepatocellular injury but rise more slowly than conjugated hyperbilirubinemia. Direct hyperbilirubinemia is the most specific, but least sensitive marker of TPNAC hepatic dysfunction/cholestasis.

The incidence of TPNAC is inversely related to gestational age and birth weight. TPNAC occurs in 50% of infants weighing less than 1000 grams at birth as compared to 7% of infants weighing more than 1500 grams at birth. Although many risk factors for development of TPNAC have been identified, cause–effect has not been clearly demonstrated for any of them. Such risk factors include prematurity, low birth weight, immature hepatobiliary system, short bowel syndrome, duration of TPN, sepsis, necrotizing enterocolitis, small bowel bacterial overgrowth, intestinal stasis, inadequate enteral nutrition, and metabolic disorders. Hermans and Teitelbaum both included protein, excessive carbohydrate and lipid, photo-oxidation products of TPN solutions, and lipid peroxidation as potential TPN hepatotoxins that may cause cholestasis in human infants. Hepatobiliary dysfunction in some infants may progress to cirrhosis, liver failure, and death. TPNAC develops in as many as 70% of infants with short bowel syndrome dependent on TPN.

## Parenteral nutrition

Excessive energy administration, or energy overloading, may contribute to TPNAC. Excessive calories, especially nonprotein calories, may cause deposition of fat within the liver and lead to hepatic dysfunction. The ideal nutrient distribution to provide energy and protein from TPN has yet to be determined for newborn infants. General guidelines for nutrient concentration, volume, amino acid and carbohydrate strategies have previously been discussed. However, it should be noted that excess glucose indirectly increases risk for cholestasis because it impairs liver function by inducing steatosis.

Furthermore, fatty acid composition in lipid emulsions varies and may impact the development of TPNAC. The parenteral lipid emulsion currently available in the United States is composed of soybean oils, primarily containing omega–6 fatty acids. Such lipid emulsions provide the preterm infant with a high concentration of calories and essential fatty acids. The phytosterols in the soybean oil have been implicated in the pathophysiology of TPNAC due to a potential harmful effect on biliary secretion and pro-inflammatory properties. It has been suggested that omega–6 fatty acids are not cleared like chylomicrons and thus accumulate in the hepatocytes. Gura et al. in 2006 reported the reversal of cholestasis in two infants with intestinal failure and TPNAC when the conventional intravenous fat-emulsion was substituted with one made from marine oil, containing primarily omega–3 fatty acids. The marine oil lipid emulsion, Omegaven™, is not currently approved by the Food and Drug Administration in the United States. It is hypothesized that intravenous omega–3 fatty acids reduce the inflammatory effect in the liver of patients with TPNAC because they are precursors for anti-inflammatory leukotrienes. The dose provided to these two preterm infants was 1 g/kg/day. Patients receiving fish-oil-based emulsions who were dependent on TPN demonstrated resolution of potentially fatal cholestatic liver disease and did not demonstrate any deleterious effects. Fat emulsions made from fish oils are promising interventions for treating and preventing TPNAC.

Other strategies to reduce the risk of TPNAC include cycling the TPN, shielding from light, and adjustment of other components, including trace elements. These strategies require more extensive investigation before being routinely implemented.

## Enteral nutrition

Enteral nutrition plays a very important role in TPNAC. TPNAC may be reversed if full enteral feeds and discontinuation of PN can be achieved before cirrhosis develops. With minimal evidence-based information available, guidelines are generally empirically determined for advancing enteral feeds in a safe and efficient manner to prevent or reverse TPNAC and avoid NEC.

## Medications

In hopes of alleviating hepatic injury caused by long-term TPN exposure and inadequate enteral nutrition, several medications and oral antibiotics may be helpful for prevention of TPNAC and advancing enteral nutrition in preterm infants. Examples of such medications include ursodiol, phenobarbital, cholecystokinin, cholestyramine, and neomycin. Ursodiol enhances bile flow and reduces the concentration of hepatotoxic bile acids. Phenobarbital is also used to induce cytochrome P-450 and to increase bile-acid-independent bile flow. Cholecystokinin improves gallbladder contractility and stimulates bile flow but there is no evidence of its efficacy in neonates. Cholestyramine is used to reduce diarrhea with SBS. Oral non-absorbable antibiotics such as gentamicin, kanamycin, neomycin and polymyxin and metronidazole are used on occasion to inhibit intestinal bacterial overgrowth. There is no consensus on the most effective antimicrobial agents.

## Conclusion

Management of preterm infants with prevention of TPNAC is challenging in patients receiving long-term TPN. Although there has not yet been an ideal TPN solution or nutritional strategy developed to reduce the incidence of TPNAC, interventions such as omega–3-containing lipid emulsions and probiotics are promising. To reduce the risk of TPNAC, Wessel and Kocoshis 2007 suggested a TPN strategy using proportional growth as the primary goal. Avoidance of excessive weight to height ratios was emphasized. The ideal long-term PN strategy to avoid TPNAC has yet to be developed.

**PRACTICAL TIPS for managing parenteral nutrition-associated cholestasis in preterm infants**

1. Limit duration of parenteral nutrition with the goal of discontinuation
2. Advance enteral feeds as tolerated with goal to meet 100% of nutritional needs
3. Use human milk as a primary source of enteral feedings; human milk should be fortified appropriately for premature infants
4. Use a pediatric-specific amino acid solution, for example: TrophAmine, Premasol, and Aminosyn PF
5. Carbohydrates to provide 40–50% of the energy supply

6. Lipids limited to 30–40% of total calories to minimize the potential for immune dysfunction and hyperlipidemia, particularly for small for gestational age or stressed neonates
7. In patients with marked progressive cholestasis associated with TPN a decrease or even a transient interruption in intravenous lipid supply may be considered
8. Copper and manganese should be monitored closely in infants with cholestasis because these trace elements are excreted through the biliary route and may be removed from TPN and provided on a weekly basis
9. Individual dosing of trace elements may be necessary in some cases of TPNAC
10. Provide adequate electrolyte, vitamin and mineral levels
11. Supplementation of pediatric multivitamin solutions which include vitamin K, and trace element solutions including copper, zinc, chromium, manganese, and selenium should be provided (with attention paid to copper and magnesium)
12. If the transaminases, alkaline phosphatase or conjugated bilirubin continue to increase, consider adding ursodeoxycholic acid

## SUGGESTED READING

Blau J, Sridhar S, Mathieson S, Chawla A. Effects of protein/ nonprotein caloric intake on parenteral nutrition-associated cholestasis in premature infants weighing 600–1000 grams. *JPEN* 2007; **31**(6):487.

Btaiche IF, Khalidi N. Parenteral nutrition-associated liver complications in children. *Pharmacotherapy* 2002; **22**(2):188.

Gura K, Duggan CP, Collier SB, et al. Reversal of parenteral nutrition-associated liver disease in two infants with short bowel syndrome using parenteral fish oil: implications for future management. *Pediatrics* 2006; **118**:197.

Hermans D. Parenteral nutrition associated liver disease. *www.Pedihepa.org* 2000; 54.

Javid PJ, Collier S, Richardson D, et al. The role of enteral nutrition in the reversal of parenteral nutrition-associated liver dysfunction in infants. *J Pediatr Surg* 2005; **40**:1015.

Kaufman SS, Gondolesi GE, Fishbein TM. Parenteral nutrition associated liver disease. *Semin Neonatol* 2003; **8**:375.

Kocoshis SA, Beath SV, Booth IW, et al. Intestinal failure and small bowel transplantation, including clinical nutrition: working group report of the second world congress of pediatric gastroenterology, hepatology, and nutrition. *J Pediatr Gastroenterol Nutr* 2004; **39**:S655.

Koletzko B, Goulet O, Hunt J, Krohn K, Shamir R. Guidelines on paediatric parenteral nutrition of the European Society of Paediatric Gastroenterology, Hepatology and Nutrition (ESPGHAN) and the European Society for Clinical Nutrition and Metabolism (ESPEM), supported by the European Society of Paediatric Research (ESPR). *J Pediatr Gastroenterol Nutr* 2005; **41**:S1.

Kubota A, Yonekura T, Hoki M, Oyanagi H, Kawahara H, et al. Total parenteral nutrition-associated intrahepatic cholestasis in infants: 25 years' experience. *J Pediatr Surg* 2000; **35**(7):1049.

Suchy, FJ. Neonatal cholestasis. *Pediatr Rev* 2004; **25**:388.

Teitelbaum DH, Drongowski R, Spivak D. Rapid development of hyperbilirubinemia in infants with the short bowel as a correlate to morbidity: possible indication for early small bowel transplantation. *Transplant Proc* 1996; **28**:2699.

Teitelbaum DH, Tracy T. Parenteral nutrition-associated cholestasis. *Semin Pediatr Surg* 2001; **10**:72.

Wessel JJ, Kocoshis SA. Nutritional management of infants with short bowel syndrome. *Semin Perinatol* 2007; **31**:104.

# Chapter 12

# Enteral nutrition

"NECiphobia" (the fear of NEC) is the most prevalent reason
clinicians withhold enteral feedings in VLBW infants. NEC
most frequently occurs in VLBW infants who have received
enteral nutrition. When parenteral nutrition is used exclusively
for the provision of nutrients, the absence of enteral feedings
is associated with morphologic and functional changes in the
gut with a significant decrease in intestinal mass, a decrease in
mucosal enzyme activity, and an increase in gut permeability.
The changes are due primarily to the lack of luminal nutrients
rather than the TPN. Therefore, parenteral nutrition does
little to support the function of the gastrointestinal tract.
The timing of the initial feedings for the preterm infant
remains controversial. As pediatric TPN solutions designed
for neonates became available, many clinicians chose to
use parenteral nutrition exclusively in the sick, ventilated,
preterm infant because of concerns about necrotizing
enterocolitis. Total parenteral nutrition was thought to be a
logical continuation of the transplacental nutrition the infants
received in utero. However, this view discounts any role that
swallowed amniotic fluid may play in nutrition and in the
development of the gastrointestinal tract. In fact, by the end
of the third trimester, the amniotic fluid provides the fetus

with the same enteral volume intake and approximately 25% of the enteral protein intake as that of a term, breastfed infant. Studies in animals maintained in an anabolic state with TPN, but deprived of enteral substrate, confirmed that intraluminal nutrition was necessary for the development of normal gastrointestinal structure and functional integrity. Enteral feedings have both direct trophic effects and indirect effects secondary to the release of intestinal hormones. Lucas et al. demonstrated significant rises in plasma concentrations of enteroglucagon, gastrin, and gastric-inhibiting polypeptide in preterm infants after milk feeds of as little as 12 mL/kg/day. Similar surges in these trophic hormones do not occur in intravenously nourished infants.

The etiology of NEC remains unclear, and is certainly multifactorial. Since NEC rarely occurs in infants who are not being fed, enteral feedings are thought to be a primary factor in the etiology of NEC. However, two issues continue to be discussed. Infants who develop NEC are more likely premature, have been enterally fed and the enteral feedings have been advanced "too fast." The association between feedings and NEC is likely to be explained by the fact that feedings act as vehicles for the introduction of bacteria, or the substrates are involved. When deciding to begin enteral nutrition in these infants, there are four fundamental questions to consider. When should enteral feedings be initiated? What type of milk should be used? Should a period of minimal enteral nutrition (MEN) be provided? How rapidly should the volume be increased? Therefore, efforts aimed at minimizing the risk of NEC have focused on the time of introduction of feedings, the diet, feeding volumes, and the rate of feeding volume increments. These strategies that had been developed with the aim of reducing the risk of NEC were shown to be ineffective. Yet "NECiphobia" continues to influence our approach to the enteral feeding of VLBW infants.

One of the main early strategies to prevent NEC involved the withholding of feeding for prolonged periods. Although it was never shown in randomized controlled trials that the prolonged withholding of feedings actually prevented NEC, some form of this strategy was widely adopted in the 1970s and into the 1980s. The withholding of feedings eventually came under scrutiny and was compared in a number of controlled trials with early introduction of feedings. A systematic review of the results of these trials concluded that early introduction of feedings shortens the time to full feeds as well as the length of hospitalization and did not lead to an increase in the incidence of NEC. A controlled study involving 100 VLBW infants fed human milk confirmed these findings and found, in addition, a significant reduction of serious infections with early introduction of feedings. However, even today as earlier enteral feeding has been adopted as a sound strategy, studies still have not included large numbers of ELBW infants to be absolutely certain that there is no increased risk of NEC especially in those critically ill infants with birthweights <1000 g.

Another strategy aimed at preventing NEC has been to keep the rate increments low. The strategy was based on the findings of Anderson and Kliegman (1991), who in their retrospective analysis of 19 cases of NEC found that in infants

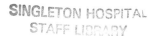
SINGLETON HOSPITAL
STAFF LIBRARY

who went on to develop NEC, feedings were advanced more rapidly than in control infants without NEC. Based on these findings, later confirmed by Berseth et al., they recommended that feedings not be advanced by more than 20 mL/kg each day. This recommendation has found wide acceptance. In a prospective randomized trial, Rayyis et al. (1999) compared increments of 15 mL/kg/d with increments of 35 mL/kg/d. They found, that with more rapid advancement, full intakes were achieved sooner, weight gain set in earlier, and there was no difference in the incidence of NEC. Limiting feeding increments in VLBW infants to 20 mL/kg/d is a standard practice. It still permits achievement of full feedings in a reasonable period (about eight days).

When initiating early enteral feedings, many ELBW infants may still have an umbilical artery catheter (UAC) in place, and controversy exists about feeding with the indwelling UAC. The presence of a UAC in small observational studies has been associated with an increased risk for NEC, and it is a common policy in many NICUs to delay feedings until catheters are removed. However, few data from controlled studies support this policy. Davey et al. (1994) examined feeding tolerance in 47 infants weighing less than 2000 g at birth who had respiratory distress and UACs. Infants were assigned randomly to begin feedings as soon as they met the predefined criterion of stability or to delay feeding until their UACs were removed for 24 hours. Infants who were fed with catheters in place started feeding significantly sooner and required half the number of days of parenteral nutrition. The incidence of NEC was comparable for infants fed with catheters in place and those whose catheters were removed before initiation of feedings. In addition, multiple large epidemiologic surveys have not shown a cause-and-effect relation between low-lying umbilical artery catheters and NEC. The question that a clinician should ask when withholding enteral feeds in an infant with a UAC is: why is the UAC in place? Is the infant critically ill? The additional clinical factors in the critically ill infant are more important in the decision to feed rather than the presence or absence of a UAC.

The decision when to start these early enteral or trophic feeds may be influenced by what milk is available to feed the infant. Lucas and Cole (1990), in a multicenter feeding trial involving almost 1000 preterm infants with birthweights less than 1850 g, demonstrated that the incidence of confirmed NEC was six times greater in formula-fed infants than in those receiving human milk that was either the infant's own mother's milk or pasteurized donor milk. In addition, NEC was rare for infants greater than 30 weeks gestation who were fed human milk, but this was not the case for formula-fed babies. A delay of feeding in the formula-fed group was associated with a reduced risk of NEC, whereas the use of early human milk feedings had no correlation with the occurrence of NEC. Therefore, initiating feeds for individual patients should take into account individual risk factors and the milk available for the patient.

Feedings should be started within the first days of life as physiologic stability is demonstrated. A frequently encountered problem is that breast milk takes several days to become available. In addition infants who are transported to distant NICUs may cause a delay in the receipt of human milk from their mothers who are still recuperating in the birth hospital. During these first days, only small amounts of colostrum are available, which is very beneficial to the infant and must be fed. Each nursery should establish criteria for feeding readiness, and agree when to consider the introduction of trophic or enteral feedings. The following list modified from the Davey et al. (1994) article is a helpful template for such consensus-building:

- Normal blood pressure and pH
- $PaO_2 > 55$
- At least 12 hours from last surfactant or indomethacin or ibuprofen dose
- Fewer than two desaturation episodes ($SaO_2$ less than 80%) per hour

Initial feeding volumes are suggested by birthweight categories. Incremental advances should be about 20 mL/kg/d when a decision is made to advance feedings

Clearly, one of the important benefits of using TPN is that it allows feedings to be advanced slowly, which probably increases the safety of enteral feedings. However, neonatologists' feeding approach to VLBW neonates has traditionally been based on local practices and not subjected to rigorous scientific investigation.

Regardless of the feeding strategy, the advancement of feedings is based on the absence of significant pregavage residuals or greenish aspirates in many NICUs. According to Ziegler and others, gastric residuals are very frequent in the early neonatal period and are virtually always benign, e.g., not associated with NEC. A recent study demonstrated that in ELBW infants, excessive gastric residual volume (GRV) either determined by percent of the previous feed or an absolute volume (>2 mL or >3 mL) did not necessarily affect feeding success as determined by the volume of total feeding reached by day 14 on a standard feeding schedule for all the study infants. Similarly the color of the GRV (green, milky, clear) did not predict feeding intolerance. Nonetheless, the volume of feeding on day 14 did correlate with a higher proportion of episodes of zero GRVs and with predominantly milky gastric residuals. Thus, isolated findings related to gastric emptying alone should not be the sole criterion in initiating or advancing feeds. Stooling pattern, abdominal distension and other clinical signs as well as the nature and frequency of stools as feedings are advanced are more important than isolated findings of GRV.

Gastric residuals therefore are normal in the first two weeks of life and are sometimes green or yellow. By themselves they do not indicate NEC or impending NEC, except when other signs are present. They tend to persist until meconium is passed and we might even consider gastric residuals as having a "protective" function as they serve as markers of gut maturation.

Given the lack of good evidence for preventing NEC, certain practices have emerged that are "conservative" in nature. For example, it is generally considered safe to begin trophic feeding within five days after birth with human milk if possible, thereafter increasing the volume of feeds as tolerated in steps of 10–20 mL/kg/d. Although NEC is a devastating complication, it only occurs in approximately 5% of VLBW infants. These conservative strategies are applied to all VLBW infants. The adverse consequences of delayed or slow advancement of enteral feeding may include prolonged use of TPN, increased risk of metabolic complications, infections and delayed hospital discharge. Since conservative feeding strategies may result in other "competing outcomes," as listed above, it is essential that future trials are powered and structured to assess the effect on long-term survival and neurodisability rates.

---

**PRACTICAL TIPS for enteral nutrition:**

1. MEN refers to small amounts of enteral feedings of formula and/or breast milk intakes <25 mL/kg/d
2. Any situation associated with gut hypoxia or decreased intestinal blood flow may contraindicate using MEN:
   Asphyxia
   Hypoxemia
   Hypotension
   Concomitant use of indomethacin or ibuprofen
3. Start MEN by day one or two. No studies have specifically addressed the optimal day to start in terms of safety and efficacy. Defining and then waiting for physiologic stability is a reasonable approach
4. Nutrition advances of ≤20 mL/kg/d do not increase the incidence of NEC
5. Breast milk is the optimal enteral feeding

6. Dilute formulas and dilute human milk fail to provide sufficient energy intake and they fail to stimulate motor activity of the GI tract. Therefore diluting milk has no role
7. Slow bolus feedings (those lasting at least 30 minutes to an hour or two) may be preferable to continuous feeds, particularly in infants with feeding intolerance
8. Gastric residuals are normal in the first two weeks of life and are sometimes green or yellow
9. Gastric residuals do not indicate NEC, or impending NEC, except when other signs of NEC are present
10. Gastric residuals may have a protective function and serve as markers of gut maturation and help you to advance feeding volumes

## SUGGESTED READING

Adamkin DH. Pragmatic approach to in-hospital nutrition in high-risk neonates. *J Perinatol* 2005; **25**(suppl):S7.

Anderson DM, Kliegman RM. The relationship of neonatal alimentation practices to the occurrence of endemic necrotizing enterocolitis. *Am J Perinatol* 1991; **8**:62.

Berseth CL. Prolonging small feeding volumes in early life decreases the incidence of necrotizing enterocolitis in very low birth weight infants. *Pediatrics* 2003; **111**:529.

Brown EG, Sweet AY. Preventing necrotizing enterocolitis in neonates. *JAMA* 1978; **240**:2452.

Caeton AJ, Goetzman BW. Risky business, umbilical arterial catheterization. *Am J Dis Child* 1985; **139**:120.

Chauhan M, Henderson G, McGuire W. Enteral feeding for very low birth weight infants: reducing the risk of necrotizing enterocolitis. *Arch Dis Child Fetal Neonatal Ed* 1993; F162–166.

Davey AM, Wagner CL, Cox C, Kendig JW. Feeding premature infants while low umbilical artery catheters are in place: a prospective, randomized trial. *J Pediatr* 1994; **124***:795.

Flidel-Rimon O, Friedman S, Lev E, et al. Early enteral feeding and nosocomial sepsis in very low birth weight infants. *Arch Dis Child Fetal Neonatal Ed* 2004; **89**:F289–292.

Kliegman RM. Studies of feeding intolerance in very low birth weight infants: Definition and significance. (Commentary) *Pediatrics* 2002; **109**:516.

Lucas A, Bloom SR, Aynsley-Green A. Gut hormones and "minimal enteral feeding." *Acta Pediatr Scand* 1986; **75**:719.

Lucas A, Cole TJ. Breast milk and neonatal necrotizing enterocolitis. *Lancet* 1990; **336**:1519.

Mihatsch WA, von Schoenaich P, Fahnenstich H, et al. The significance of gastric residuals in the early enteral feeding advancement of extremely low birth weight infants. *Pediatrics* 2002; **109**:457.

Rayyis SF, Ambalavanan N, Wright L, et al. Randomized trial of "slow" versus "fast" feed advancements on the incidence of NEC in very low birth weight infants. *J Pediatr* 1999; **134**:293–297.

Ziegler EE, Thureen PJ, Carlson SJ. Aggressive nutrition of the very-low-birth weight infant. *Clin Perinatol* 2002; **29**:225–244.

# Chapter 13

# Enteral feeding guidelines practicum

## Feeding pathways for preterm infants

### Aims

(1) To begin minimal enteral/trophic or nutritional enteral feedings, optimally, by DOL 1–2 after physiologically stable unless contraindications exist

(2) To advocate the use of human breast milk as the definitive first choice for feeds

(3) To advance feeds in a safe, yet more standardized fashion

(4) To provide guidelines for stopping feeds and identifying feeding intolerance

### Enteral feeding initiation

#### Contraindications

Hemodynamic instability

(1) Requiring volume resuscitation

(2) Pressors to maintain normal blood pressure for age

(3) Initiation of hydrocortisone especially in conjuction with indomethacin. Feeding should be delayed until hemodynamically stable for 24–48 hours. Patients may be

started on feeds while on a weaning course of
treatment of hydrocortisone if patient is hemodynamically
stable

(4) Hemodynamically significant PDA requiring
indomethacin or ibuprofen treatment or surgical
closure

- Consider feeding delay until after indomethacin and
  ibuprofen course completed or PDA ligation surgery
  completed

(5) Abnormal GI exam

- Abdominal distension, signs of obstruction, abdominal
  discoloration consistent with peritonitis, or surgical
  abdomen

(6) Signs of GI dysfunction

- Large volume gastric fluid, newly discovered discolored
  (e.g. bilious) gastric fluid

(7) Sepsis/suspect sepsis, severe metabolic acidosis, hypoxia
or hypoxemia

- Feeding should be delayed based on clinical evaluations
  in these situations

## Enteral feed choice

– Mother's breastmilk (MBM) is the feeding of choice

- MBM should be encouraged unless contraindications for
  use exist
- The substantial benefits of breast milk for the preterm
  infant, and the importance of mother's contribution,
  should be emphasized

- Breast pumping and hand expression should be initiated within the first six postpartum hours
- The value of colostrum should be emphasized – fresh colostrum should be collected and used in first feeds.
- Lactation consultations should occur, ideally, on DOL 1, or when mother is available (i.e., in cases where baby has been transferred from another hospital)

– If MBM is not available, donor breast milk (DBM) can be an alternative

- The mother/parents of VLBW infants who are not going to provide own mother's milk should be given information reviewing the benefits of human milk at the time of the "first update"

## Formula

– If formula is used, a 24 kcal/oz premature infant formula should be provided
– However, some clinicians prefer to start with a 20 kcal/oz premature infant formula; no data exist to support this practice

Tables 13.1–13.6 provide guidance for trophic and nutritional feeding for the VLBW infant. Figure 13.1 is an algorithm for management of gastric residuals in the VLBW infants.

## Colostrum use in preterm infants

- If the infant is ready to begin trophic feeds, colostrum may be administered in trophic feeds in the pathway described above

**Table 13.1** Trophic and advancing nutritional enteral feeding guidelines: feeding practice guidelines for infants < 750 g

---

*I. Trophic feedings for infants < 750 g*

| | |
|---|---|
| Initiation of feeding | Feedings start at 48 hrs of life and continue for 48 to 72 hrs |
| Feeding method | Indwelling nasogastric tube |
| Type of feeding | Expressed own mother's breast milk, donor milk or PTF24 |
| Amount of feeding | 1 mL q 4 hr (equals ~12 mL/kg/d for 500 g infant) |
| Feeding advance | None |

*II. Guide to feedings for infants <750 g*

| | |
|---|---|
| Initiation of feeding | Initiation after trophic feedings on day 5 to 6 of life |
| Feeding method | Indwelling nasogastric tube |
| Type of feeding | Expressed own mother's breast milk, donor milk or PTF24 |
| Amount of feeding | 1 mL q 2 hrs (equals an increase from trophic feeds of 12 mL/kg/d for 500 g infant) |
| Feeding advance | 1 mL/feeding q 24 hrs fortify with Pro I act +4 at 80 mL/kg/d or powdered human milk fortifiers[a] (SHMF or EHMF) at 100 mL/kg/d; continue same increase until full feeds 150–160 mL/kg/d (equals ~ 24 mL/kg/d increase for 500 g infant) |

---

[a] SHMF: Similac Human Milk Fortifier (Ross Labs, Columbus, OH).
EHMF: Enfamil Human Milk Fortifier (Mead Johnson, Evansville, IN).
Prolact +: Human Milk Fortifier (Prolacta Bioscience, Monrovia, CA).
Adapted from Premjis, Cheselli, et al. Feeding Practice Guidelines for Infants Less than 1500 grams: A before after matched cohort study. *Advances in Neonatal Care* **2**(1): 27–36, 2002. With permission.

**Table 13.2**  Feeding pathway: trophic and nutrition feeds < 750 g

| Day of feeding | mL[a] | Feedings/day (q¹) | | | mL/day |
|---|---|---|---|---|---|
| 1 | 1 | × | 6 | = | 6 |
| 2 | 1 | × | 6 | = | 6 |
| 3 | 1 | × | 6 | = | 6 |
| | *Nutritional feeding (q²)* | | | | |
| 4 | 1 | × | 12 | = | 12 |
| 5 | 2 | × | 12 | = | 24 |
| 6 | 3 | × | 12 | = | 36 |
| 7 | 4 | × | 12 | = | 46 |
| 8 | 5 | × | 12 | = | 60[b] |
| 9 | 6 | × | 12 | = | 72[b] |
| 10 | 7 | × | 12 | = | 84 |
| 11 | 8 | × | 12 | = | 96 |
| 12 | 9 | × | 12 | = | 108 |
| 13 | 10 | × | 12 | = | 120 |
| 14 | 11 | × | 12 | = | 132 |
| 15 | 12 | × | 12 | = | 144 |
| 16 | 13 | × | 12 | = | 156 |

[a]Actual increase in quantity of feeding, not based on weight.
[b]Fortify @ ~80 mL/kg/d or 100 mL/kg/d.

| | *or Nutritional feeding (q3)* | | | | |
|---|---|---|---|---|---|
| 4 | 1.5 | × | 8 | = | 12 |
| 5 | 3.0 | × | 8 | = | 24 |
| 6 | 4.5 | × | 8 | = | 36 |
| 7 | 6.0 | × | 8 | = | 48 |
| 8 | 7.5 | × | 8 | = | 60[b] |
| 9 | 9.0 | × | 8 | = | 72[b] |
| 10 | 10.5 | × | 8 | = | 84 |

**Table 13.2** (*cont.*)

| Day of feeding | mL[a] | Feedings/day (q[t]) | | | mL/day |
|---|---|---|---|---|---|
| 11 | 12.0 | × | 8 | = | 96 |
| 12 | 13.5 | × | 8 | = | 108 |
| 13 | 15.0 | × | 8 | = | 120 |
| 14 | 16.5 | × | 8 | = | 132 |
| 15 | 18.0 | × | 8 | = | 144 |
| 16 | 19.5 | × | 8 | = | 156 |

[b] Fortify.

**Table 13.3.** Feeding practice guideline for infants ≥750 g and <1000 g

*III. Trophic feedings for infants ≥750 g and <1000 g*

| | |
|---|---|
| Initiation of feedings | Start at 48 hrs of life and continue for 48 to 72 hrs |
| Feeding method | Indwelling nasogastric tube |
| Type of feeding | Expressed own mother's breast milk, donor milk or PTF 24 |
| Amount and frequency | 1 mL q 2 hrs (equals ~ 16 mL/kg/d for 750 g infant) |
| Feeding advance | None |

*IV. Guide to nutritional feedings for infants ≥750 g and <1000 g*

| | |
|---|---|
| Initiation of feeding | Initiate after trophic feedings on day 5 to 6 of life |
| Feeding method | Indwelling nasogastric tube |
| Type of feeding | Expressed own mother's breast milk, donor milk or PTF24 |
| Amount and frequency | 2mL q 2 hrs (equals ~16 mL/kg/d increase for 750 g infant) |
| Feeding advance | 1mL q 24 hrs (equals ~ 16 mL/kg/d increase for 750 g infant. Fortify with Prolact +4 or powdered human milk fortifiers[a] (SHMF or EHMF) at 80 mL/kg/d and continue same increase to 150–160 mL/kg/d |

[a] SHMF: Similac Human Milk Fortifier (Ross Labs, Columbus, OH).
EHMF: Enfamil Human Milk Fortifier (Mead Johnson, Evansville, IN).
Prolact +: Human Milk Fortifier (Prolacta Bioscience, Monrovia, CA).

**Table 13.4** Feeding pathway: trophic and nutritional feeds ≥750 g and <1000 g

| Day of feeding | mL[a] | Feedings/day (q[1]) | | | mL/day |
|---|---|---|---|---|---|
| 1 | 1 | × | 12 | = | 12 |
| 2 | 1 | × | 12 | = | 12 |
| 3 | 1 | × | 12 | = | 12 |
| | *Nutritional feeding (q[2])* | | | | |
| 4 | 2 | × | 12 | = | 24 |
| 5 | 3 | × | 12 | = | 36 |
| 6 | 4 | × | 12 | = | 48 |
| 7 | 5 | × | 12 | = | 60[b] |
| 8 | 6 | × | 12 | = | 72[b] |
| 9 | 7 | × | 12 | = | 84 |
| 10 | 8 | × | 12 | = | 96 |
| 11 | 9 | × | 12 | = | 108 |
| 12 | 10 | × | 12 | = | 120 |
| 13 | 11 | × | 12 | = | 132 |
| 14 | 12 | × | 12 | = | 144 |
| 15 | 13 | × | 12 | = | 156 |

[a] Actual increase in quantity of feeding, not based on weight.

[b] Fortify @ ~80 mL/kg/d or 100 mL/kg/d.

**Table 13.5.** Nutritional feeding guideline for infants
1000 g – <1500 g

| | |
|---|---|
| Initiation of feeding | Start at 48 hrs |
| Feeding method | Indwelling nasogastric tube |
| Type of feeding | Expressed own mother's breast milk, donor milk or PTF24 |
| Amount and frequency | 2 mL q 3 hrs (equals 16 mL/kg/d for 1000 g infant) |
| Feeding advance | 1 mL q 8 (equals an increase of 24 mMc/d for 1DDDg infant). Fortify with Prolact +4 or powdered human milk fortifiers[a] (SHMF or EHMF) at 80 mL/kg/d. Advance volume to 150–160 mL/kg/d |

[a] SHMF: Similac Human Milk Fortifier (Ross Labs, Columbus, OH).
EHMF: Enfamil Human Milk Fortifier (Mead Johnson, Evansville, IN).
Prolact +: Human Milk Fortifier (Prolacta Bioscience, Monrovia, CA).

**Table 13.6.** Nutritional feedings: birthweight
1001 g – 1500 g

| Day of feeding | mL[a] | | Feedings/day (q³) | | mL/day |
|---|---|---|---|---|---|
| 1 | 2 | × | 8 | = | 16 |
| 2 | 5 | × | 8 | = | 40 |
| 3 | 8 | × | 8 | = | 64 |
| 4 | 11 | × | 8 | = | 88[b] |
| 5 | 14 | × | 8 | = | 112 |
| 6 | 17 | × | 8 | = | 136 |
| 7 | 20 | × | 8 | = | 160 |

[a] Actual increase in quantity of feedings, not based on weight.
[b] Fortify @ ~80 mL/kg/d or 100 mL/kg/d.

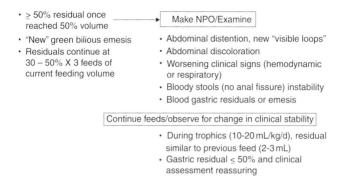

- ≥ 50% residual once reached 50% volume → Make NPO/Examine
- "New" green bilious emesis
- Residuals continue at 30 – 50% X 3 feeds of current feeding volume

- Abdominal distention, new "visible loops"
- Abdominal discoloration
- Worsening clinical signs (hemodynamic or respiratory)
- Bloody stools (no anal fissure) instability
- Blood gastric residuals or emesis

Continue feeds/observe for change in clinical stability

- During trophics (10-20 mL/kg/d), residual similar to previous feed (2-3 mL)
- Gastric residual ≤ 50% and clinical assessment reassuring

Figure 13.1  Algorithm for residuals and feeding intolerance. Adapted from personal communication with Drs. Phillip Sunshine and John Kerner, Department of Pediatrics, Stanford University.

## Feeding intolerance

- **Summary statement:** Episodes of feeding intolerance are common for preterm infants with poor peristalsis. Clinical assessment and integration of numerous pieces of information are required to ascertain the implications and importance of clinical symptoms.
- The following are *serious* signs of clinical problems and important reasons to stop feeding, consistent with possible NEC or sepsis.
  - Abdominal distention, new "visible loops," abdominal discoloration
  - Worsening clinical status, including hemodynamic or respiratory instability such as increasing bradycardias and/or apneas, poor perfusion, hypo- or hyperglycemia

  – Bloody stools not associated with anal fissure
  – Bloody gastric residual or emesis
- The following are ***potentially*** serious signs of impending or developing problems.
  – "Bilious" gastric residuals
  – A new "bilious," green or yellow residual should be assessed.
    - This finding may be associated with developing clinical problems, or may simply indicate a mechanical issue such as the orogastric tube at or beyond the pyloric sphincter.
  – "Large-volume" emesis
    - In a VLBW infant who has reached 50% of full volume feed, a large-volume emesis or residual is considered to be 50% of the last feed.
    - Other factors such as the color of the emesis, whether emesis is a new finding, changes in feeding regimen and type, and the clinical status of the infant should be assessed.
- **Gastric residuals:** The *volume of gastric residual* may or may not be indicative of looming problems. Gastric residuals should *ALWAYS* be evaluated in the context of the overall clinical assessment. Few data exist regarding the "normal" or "safe" volume of gastric residual in a feeding preterm infant.

The following should be considered GUIDELINES ONLY.

   The total volume of each feed is small, thus a gastric fluid volume equal to the total previous feed volume (2–3 mL) may be appropriate. This fluid may represent normal gastric contents. However, the quality and color of the residual, the overall clinical appearance of the infant, and whether the volumes of residuals are increasing over time should be evaluated.

- If the infant has reached >50% full feeding volume assessment is indicated when:
  - The volume of gastric residual is >30–50% of the previous
  - Residual may be discarded (×1) and feeding continued if clinical assessment is reassuring, or feeding may be held (×1)
  - The clinical assessment is not reassuring, or if > 30–50% gastric residual occurs again
  - The volume of gastric residual is < 50% and clinical assessment is reassuring, feeds may be continued
  - The residual volumes of 30–50% of feed persist for three feeds

## PRACTICAL TIPS for enteral feeding guidelines

Consider the following before making the presumption of feeding intolerance:

1. Poor positions can cause reflux. When bottle-feeding the infant should have his/her "head above the heart"

2. Medications commonly used in the NICU (antibiotics) can cause vomiting and/or diarrhea
3. Overfeeding (≥175 mL/kg) can cause vomiting or diarrhea
4. Sepsis can cause diarrhea and/or vomiting
5. CPAP can cause abdominal distention because of swallowed air
6. NG/OG tubes can cause irritation to the gut that may result in blood in the stool
7. There may be 30–50% residuals on continuous feedings. It is not necessary to check residuals on infants receiving continuous feedings
8. Preterm infants are prone to reflux. Medications or thickened formula may be used although conservative use of these medications or thickened feeds is advisable. However drugs altering gastric pH should be avoided

# Chapter 14

# Optimizing enteral nutrition: protein

There are two methods used for estimating the protein intake for ELBW infants necessary to maintain the intrauterine rate of protein accretion:

1. Factorial method, which includes an estimate of inevitable urinary nitrogen losses (i.e., the losses that occur in the absence of nitrogen intake) and an estimate of the amount deposited in utero corrected for efficiency of absorption and deposition.
2. Actual intake method, which determines the actual intake that supports intrauterine rates of growth and nitrogen accretion.

Interestingly, the two approaches do not result in the same estimate of protein requirement. The factorial method, depending on the assumptions made concerning inevitable nitrogen losses and efficiency of absorption and deposition, usually yields an estimate of approximately 4 g/kg per day to support intrauterine rates of growth and protein accretion. The actual intake method suggests that a protein intake of approximately 3 g/kg per day supports intrauterine rates of growth and nitrogen accretion.

Replicating the body composition of the fetus of the same postconceptional age as the preterm infant is as important a goal as achieving the fetal rate of weight gain. This strategy of promoting accretion of more lean mass but less fat deposition may have life-long implications. It appears with current strategies we may be promoting fat deposition and not enough lean mass. However, insufficient data are available concerning the body composition of infants fed different nutrition regimens. Furthermore, considering the marked variation in clinical practice, a targeted rate of weight gain in very preterm infants can be attained by a number of very different nutrition strategies but without consideration for "quality" of weight gain, i.e. promotion of lean mass. As nutrition regimens that produce excessive fat deposition can put the infant at risk for long-term adverse health outcomes, strategies that result in excessive fat deposition should be avoided. These regimens are sometimes used to promote growth with excessive energy in ELBW infants with postnatal growth failure. Therefore, replicating intrauterine body composition postnatally seems to be a more physiologic approach to growth in the ELBW infant. Protein and energy may be limiting factors, but especially protein needs to be provided in greater amounts than now are used. In fact, current nutritional strategies frequently provide excessive energy but not enough protein. Finally, measuring actual body compositions of very preterm infants is difficult.

Figure 14.1, adapted from Rigo and Senterre, illustrates that protein intake is the only determinant of lean body mass gain. Fat mass gain is positively related to energy intake and

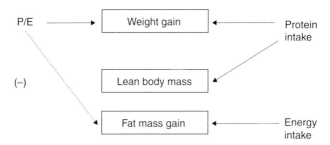

To increase LBM accretion and limit fat mass deposition, an
increase in P/E is manditory

Figure 14.1 Nutritional needs of premature infants: current
issues. Based on Rigo and Senterre (2006).

negatively to the protein/energy ratio. To increase lean mass
and limit fat mass deposition in VLBW infants, you must
increase the protein/energy ratio.

Currently, fortified human milk provides approximately
3.1 to 3.25 g of protein per 100 kcal, assuming that the human
milk has a protein content of approximately 1.4 g/100 kcal.
However, the protein content of human milk decreases with
the duration of lactation, making fortified human milk likely
to provide less protein than 3.1 to 3.25 g/100 kcal as lactation
continues. Formulas provide protein at 3–3.2 g/100 kcal. Thus,
feedings typically provide less protein (relative to energy) than
is required (at least until the infant reaches a weight of 1500 g).
This suggests that inadequate protein intake is at least partially
responsible for the poor growth of VLBW infants. Protein
should be considered the principal limiting nutrient when
considering growth in VLBW infants.

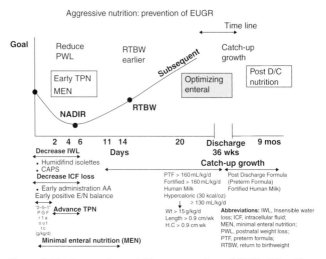

**Figure 14.2. Aggressive nutrition: prevention of EUGR.** Adamkin DH. Feeding the preterm infant. In: Bhatia J, ed. *Perinatal Nutrition Optimizing Infant Health and Development.* New York, NY: Marcel Dekker; 2004: 165–190. Reproduced with permission.

Feeding volumes must be adjusted daily to meet requirements that sustain growth of greater than 15 g/kg per day. This means providing nutrients to support not only the intrauterine rate of growth, but also "catch-up" growth (to correct deficits incurred prior to regaining birthweight). After return to birthweight the infant is more stable and catch-up growth may be accomplished (see Fig. 14.2).

Embleton and colleagues (2001) compared actual energy intake versus using an energy requirement or "goal" of 120 kcal/kg per day and documented an energy deficit of $406 \pm 92$ kcal/kg per day over the first postnatal week and a deficit of 813 ± 542 kcal/kg per day over the first 5 postnatal weeks in infants born prior to 30 weeks gestation. Interestingly, an additional 24 kcal/kg per day which would have been provided with feeding 180 mL/kg per day of preterm formula versus 150 mL/kg per day would provide an additional 840 kcal/kg over 35 days, which meets the energy deficit documented in the study. This 180 mL/kg/d would provide 4 g/kg/d of protein and 144 kcal/kg/d of energy: adequate protein but probably excessive energy to match fetal body composition.

Accordingly, preterm formula must be fed at 180 mL/kg per day during convalescence to meet protein requirements and enhance growth if the clinician is trying to reach protein at 4 g/kg/d. If feeding volumes are restricted there are numerous hypercaloric feeding strategies available allowing volume restriction while still promoting accretion of lean mass (Chapter 22).

The amino acid and energy intakes necessary to support intrauterine rates of weight gain and protein accretion, whether administered parenterally or enterally, are approximately 3 g/kg per day and approximately 90 kcal/kg per day, respectively, when matched to the early-gestation fetus (< 28 weeks). However, such intakes do not abolish any loss of lean body mass that occurred before the infant regained his or her birthweight. Accomplishing this goal requires an additional allowance for catch-up growth, which varies considerably from infant to infant. For example, the infant who does not regain birthweight until 28 days of age has twice the catch-up needs of an infant who weighs the same at birth but regains birthweight at 14 days of age. In both cases, the needs for catch-up growth are additional to the needs for supporting intrauterine rates of growth and protein accretion. These differing needs for catch-up growth make it difficult to define a single protein requirement that is appropriate for all ELBW infants; rather, each infant is likely to have a unique requirement consisting of the need for maintaining intrauterine rates of growth and protein retention (approximately 3.0 g/kg per day) plus the needs for catch-up, i.e. a total protein requirement near or even greater than 4 g/kg/d.

Currently, modern preterm formulas and supplemented human milk provide protein intakes of 3.3 to 3.6 g/kg per day at an energy intake of 120 kcal/kg per day. Once established, such intakes support growth and protein accretion rates somewhat in excess of intrauterine rates, but most infants fed these intakes remain below the 10th percentile of intrauterine standards at discharge. It is clear that most ELBW and perhaps some VLBW infants are likely to benefit from a higher protein intake. However, there is no clear evidence that an energy intake of more than 120 kcal/kg per day is desirable. A higher energy intake may promote better protein utilization, but it may result in higher rates of fat accretion. Strive for the maximal possible gain without adverse effects since the optimal gain for each infant is not known.

Table 14.1 provides new recommendations for protein and protein/energy ratio in relation to postconceptional age and the need for catch-up growth (Rigo and Senterre, 2006). The recommendations are made according to postconception age. The ability to measure lean body mass accretion and

**Table 14.1** Revised recommended protein intake and protein-energy ratio for premature infants according to postconceptional age and the need for catch-up.

|  | Without need for catch-up growth | With need for catch-up growth |
| --- | --- | --- |
| 26–30 weeks PCA:<br>16–18 g/kg/d LBM 14%<br>protein retention | 3.8–4.2 g/kg/d<br>PER: ±3.0 | 4.4 g/kg/d<br>PER: ± 3.3 |
| 30–36 weeks PCA:<br>14–15 g/kg/d LBM 15%<br>protein retention | 3.4–3.6 g/kg/d<br>PER: ±2.8 | 3.6–4.0 g/kg/d<br>PER: ± 3.0 |
| 36–40 weeks PCA:<br>13 g/kg/d LBM 17%<br>protein retention | 2.8–3.2 g/kg/d<br>PER: 2.4–2.6 | 3.CL3.4 g/kg/d<br>PER: 2.6–2.8 |

PCA, postconceptual age; LBM, lean body mass; PER, protein/energy ratio, gram of protein/100 kcal.
Data from Rigo J and Senterre J (2006) with permission. Copyright © 2006 Mosby, Inc. All rights reserved.

body composition noninvasively will be an important tool in the future.

Optimal early nutrition, both parenteral and enteral, obviously can reduce the time required to regain birthweight and, hence, reduce the protein needed to support catch-up growth. Nonetheless, most infants probably require a higher protein intake from supplemented human milk and formula rather than is currently provided. Recent recommendations reflect this likely need for a higher protein content of human milk fortifiers and preterm formulas. A committee appointed by the Life Sciences Research Organization to evaluate the nutrient contents of preterm formulas recommended a maximum protein content of 3.6 g/100 kcal, which when fed at 120 kcal/kg/d will provide 4.3 g/kg/d of protein. This recommendation and those found in Table 14.1 will provide guidance to optimize enteral nutrition for the VLBW infant.

## SUGGESTED READING

Dashyap S, Schulze KF, Ramakrishnan R, Dell RB, Heird WC. Evaluation of mathematical model for predicting the relationship between protein and energy intakes of low-weight infants and the rate and composition of weight gain. *Pediatr Res* 1994; **35**:704–712.

Embleton NE, Pang N, Cooke RJ. Postnatal malnutrition and growth retardation: an inevitable consequence of current recommendations in preterm infants? *Pediatrics* 2001; **107**:270–273.

Ernst KD, Radmacher PG, Rafail ST, et al. Postnatal malnutrition of extremely low birthweight infants with catch-up growth postdischarge. *J Perinatol* 2003; **23**:447–482.

Groh-Wargo S, Thompson M, Hovasi-Cox J. *Nutritional Care for High Risk Newborns.* 3rd ed. Chicago, IL: Bonus Books; 2000.

Klein CJ. Nutrient requirements for preterm infant formulas. *J Nutr* 2002; **132**:1395S–1577S.

Rigo J, Senterre J. Nutritional needs of premature infants: current issues. *J Pediatr* 2006; **149**:S80–88.

Thureen P, Heird WC. Protein and energy requirements of the
    preterm/low birthweight (LBW) infant. *Pediatr Res* 2005;
    **57**:95R–98R.
Ziegler EE, Thureen PJ, Carlson SJ. Aggressive nutrition of
    the very-low-birth weight infant. *Clin Perinatol* 2002;
    **29**:225–244.

SINGLETON HOSPITAL
STAFF LIBRARY

# Chapter 15

# Human milk

Although breast milk is considered the ideal food for the term infant, for the VLBW infant it provides inadequate amounts of several nutrients, especially protein, vitamin D, calcium, phosphorus, and sodium. While large volumes of human milk (180 mL/kg/d) provide the energy sufficient to enable nearly all infants with birthweights <1250 g to gain weight at intrauterine rates (approximately 15 g/kg/d), the *protein* content is suboptimal, and may result in lower serum albumin and transthyretin (prealbumin) levels, which are reliable indicators of protein nutrition in preterm infants. The calcium and phosphorus content is low in unsupplemented human milk regardless of large volumes in comparison with that required to achieve intrauterine accretion rates, resulting in poor bone mineralization in VLBW infants. In addition, the sodium content of human milk results in less sodium retention than intrauterine estimates and may result in hyponatremia and may be rate-limiting for appropriate weight gain

Lucas and colleagues (1984) found that infants weighing less than 1200 g at birth fed unfortified human milk were less than two standard deviations below the mean for weight for age when they reached 2.0 kg. Therefore, infants weighing less than 1.0 kg at birth who were fed unfortified human milk would be expected to take three weeks longer to reach a weight of 2.0 kg than infants receiving preterm formulas.

In a study focusing on developmental outcomes, Lucas et al. (1989) observed that infants receiving breast milk had a significantly higher intelligence quotient at eight years than formula-fed infants. These studies included infants receiving unfortified donor human milk. Therefore, both mother's own milk and donor human milk may confer developmental advantages. Improved visual outcomes have also been reported for human-milk-fed VLBW infants as well as for infants fed with formula containing higher levels of docosahexanoic acid (DHA) and arachidonic acid (ARA).

Human milk also has other nonnutritional advantages. For example, human milk contains immunocompetent cellular components, including secretory IgA, which has a protective effect on the intestinal mucosa. This protection and the promotion of a "healthier" colonization of bacteria in the immature gut may perhaps partially explain how human milk prevents NEC in preterm infants.

Since the composition of preterm milk varies greatly from one mother to another and the concentration of nutrients in preterm milk changes over time, it is difficult to determine the actual intake of an infant. To confer the potential nonnutritional advantages yet provide optimal nutrient intake, human milk should be supplemented, or fortified, with protein, calcium, phosphorus, vitamin D, and sodium. Infants born at ≤ 32 weeks estimated gestational age are candidates to

receive supplementation in order to prevent poor growth and
osteopenia.

There are multiple fortification strategies available and
include mixing human milk with a standard 24 kilocalorie
per ounce preterm formula producing an approximately
22 kilocalorie/ounce milk that enhances macro- and
micronutrient composition. Human milk may also be mixed
with a 30 kcal/ounce liquid formulation to produce a 24 or
25 kcal/ounce milk. The benefit of this strategy is avoidance

## Table 15.1  Human milk fortification

| Milk at 100 kilocalories | ml | Protein (g) | Fat (g) | CHO (g) | Ca (mg) | P (mg) |
|---|---|---|---|---|---|---|
| PTHM | 150 | 2.1 | 5.8 | 9.9 | 37 | 19 |
| *24 kcal/ounce* | | | | | | |
| PTHM + SSC30 4:3 ratio | 125 | 2.6 | 6.2 | 8.7 | 113 | 62 |
| PTHM + SHMF 1 pkt/25 mL | 125 | 3.0 | 5.2 | 10.4 | 175 | 98 |
| PTHM + EHMF 1 pkt/25 mL | 125 | 2.9 | 5.9 | 8.7 | 121 | 66 |
| PTHM + SSC30 1:1 ratio | 120 | 2.7 | 6.1 | 9.0 | 122 | 68 |
| *25 kcal/ounce* | | | | | | |
| Prolact+4 | 100 | 2.3 | 4.9 | 7.3 | 128 | 70 |

PTHM, preterm human milk, 1.5 g protein/100 mL.

SSC30, Similac Special Care (Abbott Nutrition, Columbus, OH).

EHMF, Enfamil Human Milk Fortifier (Mead Johnson, Evansville, IN).

Prolact+4, Prolacta Biosciences, Monrovia, CA.

SHMF, Similac Human Milk Fortifier.

of powders that are not sterile. However, the disadvantages include diluting the amount of human milk fed to the infant and concerns that the "mixing" may decrease the benefit of the human milk. Two powdered human milk fortifiers, EHMF and SHMF, may be added to make 22 or 24 kilocalorie/ounce fortified human milk. There is now a fortifier made from human milk to make a 24 kilocalorie/ounce human milk (Prolacta +4). All these fortifiers are shown in Table 15.1. Chapters 20 and 22 on calcium and phosphorus and hypercaloric feedings respectively also address human milk fortification strategies.

---

### PRACTICAL TIPS for human milk

The lactation consultant should meet the mother as soon as she is available and the health care team should enthusiastically support the acquisition and use of human milk in the NICU and post-discharge

Preferable to feed human milk intermittently rather than continuous drip method. Syringe should be inverted to prevent "creaming out" of fat and loss of up to 30% of energy to tubing with continuous infusion of human milk

Human milk fortification for all infants ≤ 32 weeks EGA, <1500 g birthweight.

Human milk fortified with powders may be fortified when the infant achieves an enteral intake of 80–100 mL/kg/d

Human milk fortified with a donor human milk fortifier can be fortified at even lower volumes

## SUGGESTED READING

Carlson SJ, Ziegler EE. Nutrient intakes and growth of very low birth weight infants. *J Perinatol* 1998; **18**:252–258.

Kuscel CA, Harding JE. Multicomponent fortified human milk for promoting growth in preterm infants. *Cochrane Review. The Cochrane Library*; 2005.

Lucas A, Gore SM, Cole TJ, et al. Multi-centre trial on feeding low birthweight infants: effects of diet on early growth. *Arch Dis Child* 1984; **59**:722.

Lucas A, Morley R, Cole TJ, et al. Early diet in preterm babies and developmental status in infancy. *Arch Dis Child* 1989; **64**:1570.

Schanler RJ, Atkinson SA. Human milks. In: RC Tsang, B. Koletza, R Vauy and S Zlotkin, eds. *Nutrition of the Preterm Infant: Scientific Basis and Practical Guidelines*. 2nd ed. Cincinnati: Digital Educational Publishing; 2005.

# Chapter 16

# Premature infant formulas

Providing optimal nutrition to a VLBW infant is difficult because there is no natural standard for comparison. For the healthy full-term infant, human milk is considered the "gold standard." Human milk is used as the reference for the development of commercial infant formulas. While the milk of mothers who deliver their infants prematurely transiently has higher nitrogen, fatty acid content, sodium, chloride, magnesium, and iron, it is still inadequate for other nutrients, especially calcium and phosphorus. Therefore premature breast milk cannot be used as a standard for the development of premature infant formula. The special premature infant formulas use data from the accretion rates of various nutrients relative to the reference fetus, and from clinical studies of the development of the gastrointestinal tract which have defined the efficiency of absorption of nutrients and from metabolic studies.

The premature infant formulas are whey-predominant, which produces less metabolic acidosis than casein-predominant formulas in VLBW infants. The risk of lactobezoar formation is reduced when a whey-predominant formula is used. In addition, the concentration of protein per liter is approximately 50% greater than that of standard infant formula to provide three to four grams protein/kg per day (depending on volume fed). The fat is approximately 50% LCT and 50% MCT. The vitamin concentration is higher because the volume of formula consumed is significantly less in the VLBW infant. The calcium and phosphorus content is greater than standard formula, with some variation between formula manufacturers. The calcium-to-phosphorus ratio generally is 2:1 as compared to 1.4:1 to 1.5:1 with standard infant formulas. As with all formulas, it is important to shake the formula before use, because precipitation may occur and the precipitate, containing high amounts of calcium and phosphorus, may remain in the bottom of the container.

Premature infant formulas have a lower lactose concentration than term formulas (approximately 50% of the carbohydrate is lactose), which reduces the lactose load. The premature infant has a relative lactase deficiency. The remainder of the carbohydrate is provided as glucose polymers or other sugars, which are readily hydrolyzed by glucoamylase and result in a product with low osmolality.

Premature infant formulas are low in iron content (3 mg elemental iron/L) as these infants often received transfusions and since the use of iron would increase the requirement for vitamin E. However, because some infants are receiving this type of formula for greater than two months and because the advantages of continuing a baby on a nutrient-enriched formula after hospital discharge have been recognized, premature infant formulas are available both with low iron content (3 mg elemental iron/L) and with iron fortification (15 mg elemental iron/L). Some manufacturers are discontinuing the production of low-iron formulas.

The sodium content of premature infant formula is greater than that of both human milk and standard infant formula.

Sodium requirements vary considerably between infants, so this amount may be inadequate to maintain normal serum levels, particularly in infants receiving diuretics. Supplementation with sodium chloride may be necessary. One distinct advantage of premature infant formula is that, despite the high concentration of nutrients, the 24 kilocalorie/oz premature infant formula is iso-osmolar, with osmolalities ranging from 280 to 300 mOsm/kg $H_2O$.

As discussed in the chapter on human milk, preterm infants provided human milk have advanced visual and neurodevelopmental outcome as compared to formula-fed infants, measured by electroretinograms, visual evoked potentials, and psychometric tests. The better performance has been related to dietary DHA and ARA acids, since plasma and erythrocyte phospholipid contents of ARA and DHA are higher in breast-fed infants than in infants fed formulas lacking these fatty acids. Therefore there may be an association between inadequate long-chain fatty acids in the diet and performance on tests of vision and cognitive function. The inability to synthesize enough DHA and ARA from their precursors and the lack of preformed DHA explain the lower blood levels of these fatty acids in formula-fed infants. The recent addition of these fatty acids to formulas in the United States has led to renewed interest and debate about the effects of long-chain fatty acids on later neurodevelopmental outcome. It should be emphasized that human milk DHA content differs among women and declines during lactation. Therefore, supplementation of breast-feeding mothers with DHA has been recommended and some studies demonstrate benefit to the infant as late as

3–5 years after supplementation of the mother for a few weeks postpartum.

The composition of the commercially available formulas for preterm infants in the United States are shown in Table 16.1. The higher-density formula (101 kcal/100 mL) may

**Table 16.1** Macronutrient and mineral composition of available preterm infant formulas

| Component (amount/120 kcal) | Similac Special Care Advance® 20 and 24 | Enfamil Premature andLipil® 20 and 24 | Similac Special Care Advance® 30 |
|---|---|---|---|
| Protein (g)[a] | 3.6 | 3.6 | 3.6 |
| Carbohydrate (g) | 12.4 | 13.2 | 9.2 |
| Lactose (g) | 6.2 | 5.3 | 4.6 |
| Fat (g) | 6.5 | 6.1 | 7.9 |
| MCT (g) | 3.25 | 2.44 | 3.95 |
| LA (mg) | 840 | 972 | 840 |
| ALA (mg) | 133 | 144 | 133 |
| ARA (mg)[b] | 26.1 | 40.8 | 26.1 |
| DHA (mg)[b] | 16.3 | 20.4 | 16.3 |
| Calcium (mg) | 216 | 198 | 216 |
| Phosphorus (mg) | 120 | 100 | 120 |

MCT, medium-chain triglycerides; LA, linoleic acid; ALA, alpha-linolenic acid; ARA, arachidonic acid; DHA, docosahexaenoic acid.

[a] Protein content of the formulas is composed of bovine milk and whey proteins with a 60:40 ratio of whey proteins:caseins.

[b] Both formulas have less than 0.5% of C. cohnii oil and M. alpine oil as source of docosahexaenoic acid (DHA) and arachidonic acid (ARA).

From Kashyap S. Enteral intake for very low birth weight infants: what should the composition be? In: RA Ehrenkranz and BB Poindexter, eds. *Seminars in Perinatology*, vol 31, No 2, 2007. With permission from Elsevier.

be used to increase the nutrient density of the feeding regimens and can also be mixed with 81 kcal/100 mL formula to provide 87–95 kcal/100 mL milk without increasing the fluid volume. It can also be used as a ready-to-feed formula providing 30 kcal/30 mL. This formula has increased fat and lower carbohydrate content, but also the osmolality and potential renal solute load are higher (325 mOsm/kg water and 28.2/100 mL versus 280 mOsm/kg, water and 22.6/100 mL respectively). Strategies with hypercaloric milks like this one will be discussed in Chapter 22.

We do not recommend using a high-energy-density formula as a ready-to-feed formula early when feeds are being established in VLBW infants.

---

### PRACTICAL TIPS for premature infant formulas

Indication for premature 24 kilocalorie per ounce formula

Weight is ≤ 1800 grams

≤ 34 weeks EGA

No human milk available

Used to supplement human milk

---

### SUGGESTED READING

Birch DG, Birch EE, Hoffman DR, Uauy RD. Retinal development in very-low-birth-weight infants fed diets differing in omega–3 fatty acids. *Invest Ophthalmol Vis Sci* 1992; **33**:2365.

Birch EE, Birch DG, Hoffman DR, Uauy RD. Dietary essential fatty acid supply and visual acuity development. *Invest Ophthalmol Vis Sci* 1992; **32**:3242.

Jensen CL, Heird WC. Lipids with an emphasis on long-chain polyunsaturated fatty acids. *Clin Perinatol* 2002; **29**:261.

O'Connor DL, Hall R, Adamkin D, et al. Growth and development in preterm infants fed long chain polyunsaturated fatty acids: a prospective randomized control trial. *Pediatrics* 2007; **108**:359–371.

# Chapter 17

# Standard Infant Formulas

Term infant formulas do not meet the nutritional requirements for VLBW infants. Yet many preterm babies may be discharged on term formulas and some even receive them in the NICU. The carbohydrate in standard infant formula is 100% lactose and the fat is all long-chain triglycerides of vegetable origin, usually soy and coconut oils. Most standard formulas are whey-predominant, with 60% of the protein whey and 40% casein. Standard formulas are available in both iron-fortified and non-iron-fortified (or "low iron") forms. Iron-fortified formula contains elemental iron 12 mg/L or approximately 2.0 mg/kg per day for an infant receiving approximately 108 kcal/kg/d. Low-iron formula contains elemental iron 1.5 mg/L or 0.2 mg/kg per day.

Most standard infant formulas are available as ready-to-feed, liquid concentrate, and powder. The concentrate and the powder provide the option of concentrating the formula to a higher caloric density. Concentrations above 1 kilocalorie per milliliter or 30 kilocalories per ounce are not recommended because of the high renal solute load that results from the decrease in free water intake. As the formula is concentrated, the osmolality increases to approximately the same degree as the concentration. Thus, for a 20 kcal/oz formula with an

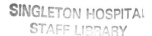
SINGLETON HOSPITAL
STAFF LIBRARY

osmolality of 300 mOsm/kg $H_2O$, if concentrated 135% or to a 27 kcal/oz formula, the osmolality increases to approximately 405 mOsm/kg $H_2O$. This concentration of term formula is not an accepted strategy for nutrient-enhancing a VLBW infant in the NICU. The chapter on hypercaloric feeding strategies (Chapter 22) discusses acceptable milks where overconcentrating is not a likely hazard for small preterm infants.

Standard term formulas do not support catch-up growth as well because of lower protein content and less calcium and phosphorus vs. post-discharge formulas for those infants discharged on formula. The basic composition of a term formula is shown in comparison with a post-discharge formula in Chapter 25.

---

### PRACTICAL TIPS for standard infant formulas

1. Standard cow-milk-based formulas are designed to mimic the nutrient content of human milk
2. These formulas contain 20 kilocalories per ounce and are appropriate for most term infants
3. Indications include:
   Birthweight $\geq$ 2500 grams
   EGA $\geq$ 37 weeks
   Human milk not available
   Protein and caloric needs can be met with a standard term 20 kilocalorie per ounce formula
4. Not indicated for VLBW infants during hospitalization or after discharge

# Chapter 18

# Soya formulas

The isolated soy-based formulas on the USA market are free of cow's milk protein and lactose. The soy protein is a soy isolate supplemented with L-methionine, L-carnitine and taurine. Soy-based formulas are not designed to meet the nutritional needs of the premature infant. These are not recommended because of the low calcium and phosphorus content of these formulas as well as generally not meeting the nutritional requirements for VLBW infants. Preterm infants fed soy protein formulas have significantly lower serum phosphorus and serum alkaline phosphatase levels and an increased risk of development of osteopenia. Even when supplemented with additional calcium, phosphorus, and vitamin D, VLBW infants fed these formulas exhibit slower weight gain and lower serum protein and albumin concentrations than infants receiving a whey-predominant premature infant formula.

## SUGGESTED READING

Bhatia J, Greer FR. The use of soy protein based formulas in infant feeding. *Pediatrics* 2008; **121**:1062–1068.

O'Connor DL, Brennan J. Formulas for preterm and term infants In: P Thureen and WW Hay, eds. *Neonatal Nutrition and Metabolism*. Cambridge University Press; 2006.

# Chapter 19

# Protein hydrolysate formulas

Protein hydrolysate formulas are designed for infants who
are allergic to cow's milk or soy proteins. Some protein
hydrolysate formulas are also elemental with the carbohydrate
in easily absorbable forms, such as glucose polymers or
monosaccharides, and the fat as both medium-chain and
long-chain triglycerides. These are sometimes used in the
management of infants with intestinal resection or intractable
diarrhea. These formulas can be loosely categorized according
to the extent that the protein is hydrolyzed: (1) 100% free
amino acid-containing formula (SHS Neocate); (2) extensively
hydrolyzed protein-containing formula (Enfamil Nutramigen,
Enfamil Pregestimil, Similac Alimentum); and (3) partially
hydrolyzed protein-containing formula (Carnation Good Start)
(Table 19.1).

All of these protein hydrolysate formulas provide
67–68 kcal/dL energy. These formulas are not routinely
recommended for VLBW infants but are used frequently in
VLBW infants after intestinal resection resulting from NEC. A
recent review by Szajewska concluded there was little evidence
to support the use of extensive and partial protein hydrolysate
formulas for preterm infants.

**Table 19.1** Macronutrient content of protein hydrolysate-based formulas and amino acid formation[a]

| | Enfamil Pregestimil | Similac Alimentum | Enfamil Nutramigen | SHS Neocate |
|---|---|---|---|---|
| Protein (g 100 kcal⁻¹) | 2.8 | 2.75 | 2.8 | 3.7 amino acids, 3.1 g protein equivalent |
| Protein source | Hydrolyzed casein with added cystine, tyrosine, tryptophan, and taurine | Hydrolyzed casein with added cystine, tyrosine, tryptophan and taurine | Hydrolyzed casein with added cystine, tyrosine, tryptophan and taurine | 100% free amino acids including taurine and carnitine |
| Carbohydrate (g 100 kcal⁻¹) | 10.2 | 10.2 | 10.3 | 11.7 |
| Carbohydrate sources | Corn syrup solids, modified corn starch, +/− dextrose | Sucrose +/− modified tapioca starch, +/− corn maltodextrin | Corn syrup solids and modified corn starch | Corn syrup solids |
| Fat (g 100 kcal⁻¹) | 5.6 | 5.5 | 5.3 | 4.5 |
| Fat sources[b] | 55% MCT oil, soy oil, corn oil, high oleic safflower, sunflower oil | 33% MCT oil, safflower oil, soy oil | Palm olein oil, soy oil, coconut oil, high oleic sunflower oil | High oleic coconut oil (5% as MCT), soy oil |

[a] See www.meadjohnson.com, www.ross.com and www.shsna.com for the most recent product information.

[b] Inclusion of single cell oils is being phased in at the time of writing. Fat blends may differ depending on whether a concentrate, ready-to-feed or powder.

From O'Connor DL and Brennan J. Formulas for preterm and term infants. In: Thureen PJ and Hay WW, eds. *Neonatal Nutrition and Metabolism*, second edition. Cambridge University Press, 2006.

## SUGGESTED READING

O'Connor DL, Brennan J. Formulas for preterm and term
infants. In: P Thureen and WW Hay, eds. *Neonatal Nutrition
and Metabolism.* Cambridge University Press; 2006.

Scajewska H. Extensive and partial protein hydrolysate
preterm formula. *J Pediatr Gastroenterol Nutr* 2007;
**45**:S183–188.

# Chapter 20

# Enteral calcium, phosphorus, magnesium, and vitamin D

The amount of enteral calcium, phosphorus, and magnesium intake required to match intrauterine accretion rates is high: calcium 185 to 200 mg/kg per day, phosphorus 100 to 113 mg/kg per day, and magnesium 5.3 to 6.1 mg/kg per day. VLBW infants with a less complicated clinical course may require lower intakes. The American Academy of Pediatrics recommends intakes of calcium of 185 to 210 mg/kg per day, phosphorus 123 to 140 mg/kg per day, and magnesium 8.5 to 10.0 mg/kg per day. However, magnesium intake at this level with such high calcium and phosphorus intake results in negative magnesium balance; therefore, a higher intake of magnesium approximately 20 mg/kg per day may be needed.

The recommendation for vitamin D, which is required for normal metabolism of calcium, phosphorus, and magnesium, has ranged from 200 to 2000 IU per day for the preterm infant. VLBW infants can maintain normal vitamin D status with 400 IU per day. Providing high-dose vitamin D supplementation does not decrease the incidence of osteopenia in VLBW infants.

Human milk has concentrations of calcium and phosphorus that are appropriate for full-term infants. These amounts are inadequate for the VLBW infant. Breast milk should be supplemented with additional calcium, phosphorus, and vitamin D, which can easily be done with a powdered human milk fortifier (Enfamil Human Milk Fortifier, Mead Johnson, Evansville, IN; Similac Human Milk Fortifier, Abbott Laboratories, Columbus, OH). Also recently available is a human milk fortifier (Prolact + H$^2$MF, Prolacta, Bioscience, Monrovia, CA). Fortification yields better mineral accretion than breast milk alone, similar to that of VLBW infants fed a premature infant formula. Although both available preterm formulas have calcium and phosphorus carbonate as the source of calcium and phosphorus, Enfamil premature formula Lipil® also has added calcium chloride and calcium hydroxide. Soluble calcium may result in greater net absorption, but may decrease fat absorption. Only relatively insoluble salts (calcium phosphate and calcium carbonate) are used in Similac®, whereas both soluble (calcium glycerophosphate and calcium gluconate) and insoluble salts (calcium phosphate) are used in the Enfamil® Human Milk Fortifier. Balance studies in VLBW infants report calcium absorption of 40 to 70% in infants fed preterm formula and 50 to 70% in those receiving a powdered fortified human milk.

As mentioned earlier, "liquid" fortification strategies to avoid the use of powders may be preferred. These strategies may not provide as much calcium and phosphorus. The content of human milks and various formulas appear in Table 20.1.

Inadequate intakes of calcium, phosphorus, and vitamin D result in metabolic bone disease of prematurity, also called rickets of prematurity or osteopenia. This disease is

**Table 20.1**  Calcium and phosphorus intake with available preterm formulas and powered human milk fortifiers (HMF) when fed at 120 kcal/kg/d[a]

|  | PTF | HMF |
|---|---|---|
| Calcium intake (mg/kg/d) | 198–216 | 173–210 |
| Phosphorus intake (mg/kg/d) | 100–120 | 95–118 |

[a] These intakes provide retention equal to intrauterine accretion rates in VLBW infants.

characterized by reduced bone mineralization and, in severe cases, frank radiologic evidence of demineralization and spontaneous fractures. The biochemical findings, although not highly sensitive, include an elevated alkaline phosphatase (>1000 U/L), decreased serum phosphorus (<4 mg/dL), and normal serum calcium. The 25-hydroxycholecalciferol (25-OH vitamin D) level is usually normal, but 1,25-dihydroxycholecalciferol (1,25-OH vitamin D) levels may be elevated as a result of increased parathyroid hormone levels and low serum phosphorus levels. The incidence of osteopenia was much higher before institution of the current nutrient practice of higher calcium and phosphorus levels in parenteral nutrient solution and early enteral feedings. The etiology of osteopenia is thought to be primarily an inadequate intake of calcium and phosphorus and the usual finding is hypophosphatemia. Risk factors for osteopenia are listed in Table 20.2.

Fortified human milk or premature infant formulas are the preferred feedings for VLBW infants. The use of soy or term

**Tabel 20.2** Risk factors for metabolic bone disease of prematurity

---

Extremely low birth weight (≤1000 g)

Prolonged parenteral nutrition

Unsupplemented human milk

Use of elemental formulas and soy formulas

Chronic diuretic therapy (especially furosemide)

Chronic problems such as necrotizing enterocolitis, bronchopulmonary dysplasia, cholestasis and acidosis

---

formulas is not recommended for infants with birthweight < 2500 g. If continuous infusion feeding of human milk is necessary, the syringe and the pump should be placed upright to prevent loss of calcium, phosphorus, and milk fat by separation and adherence to the tubing.

## SUGGESTED READINGS

Kashyap S. Enteral intake for very low birth weight infants: what should the composition be? In: RA Ehrenkranz and BB Poindexter, eds. *Semin Perinatol* 2007; **31** (2).

Mize CE, Uauy R, Waidelich D, et al. Effect of phosphorus supply on mineral balance at high calcium intakes in very low birth weight infants. *Am J Clim Nutr* 1995; **62**: 385–391

Schanler RJ, Abrams SA. Postnatal attainment of intrauterine macromineral accretion rates in low birth weight infants fed fortified human milk. *J Pediatr* 1995; **126**:441–447.

# Chapter 21

# Iron

There has been increased interest in iron deficiency, with data suggesting that mental and developmental test scores are lower in infants with iron deficiency anemia and that iron therapy sufficient to correct the anemia is insufficient to reverse the behavioral and developmental disorders in many infants. This indicates that certain ill effects are persistent depending on the timing, severity, or degree of iron-deficiency anemia during infancy.

Iron stores in the preterm infant are lower than in the term baby because these stores are relatively proportional to body weight. Iron depletion occurs at the time the infant doubles her/his birthweight and thus iron therapy should begin by two to four weeks of life in the preterm infant when enteral feedings are tolerated. VLBW infants may need as much as 4–6 mg/kg per day, with about 2 mg/kg per day provided by iron-fortified formula and the remainder as iron supplementation at 2–4 mg/kg per day. A higher dose is also necessary for infants being given erythropoietin. Although premature infant formulas, both with and without iron fortification, are manufactured with ample amounts of vitamin E and a polyunsaturated fatty acid-to-E ratio of 6.0 or greater, premature infants on human milk and receiving supplemental iron should also be supplemented with 4 to 5 mg (6 to 8 IU) of vitamin E per day. This can be readily accomplished by use of an oral multivitamin with iron.

To avoid the risk of iron toxicity related to immature antioxidant systems in VLBW infants, the AAP and other organizations do not recommend using iron prior to two weeks of age. Because of the risk of cumulative multiple red blood cell transfusions on iron status, during hospitalization, VLBW infants are at risk for iron toxicity. Low vitamin E concentrations and an immature vitamin C scavenging system the first weeks of life are responsible for immature antioxidant activity. An early oxidant challenge from iron may result in tissue damage due to unquenched free radicals.

The impression that low-iron formulas are associated with fewer gastrointestinal disturbances is not supported by controlled studies. Because the bioavailability of iron from iron-fortified infant cereals is somewhat low, it is recommended that iron-fortified formulas or daily iron supplements be continued through the first year of life.

### SUGGESTED READING

American Academy of Pediatrics, Committee on Nutrition. Iron fortification of infant formulas. *Pediatrics* 1999; **104**:119.

Georgieff MK. Iron. In: P Thureen, and WW Hay, eds. *Neonatal Nutrition and Metabolism*. 2nd ed. Cambridge University Press; 2006.

Walter T, DeAndraca I, Chadud P, et al. Iron deficiency anemia: adverse effects on infant psychomotor development. *Pediatrics* 1989; **84**:7.

# Chapter 22

# Hypercaloric feeding strategy

This strategy is intended for use in critically ill VLBW infants who cannot tolerate sufficient volume of feedings to meet their needs for growth with a standard premature formula or fortified breast milk. Until recently, various mixtures of powders and "manipulation" of milk to make concentrated formulas were used. The goal was to increase energy and increase protein intake in these fluid-restricted infants. However, attainment of adequate protein remained difficult. In addition, precise mixing was problematic and the use of powders in reconstituting these formulas had the potential for not only mixing errors but also for the introduction of microbials into those mixtures being fed to immunocompromised preterm infants. Providing enough protein is the challenge in the moderate to severely fluid-restricted infants.

The recent introduction of a 30 kilocalorie per ounce liquid ready-to-feed preterm formula (Similac Special Care Advance® 30) increases nutrient density of feeding regimens without increasing the fluid volume. Therefore the mixing of powdered formula and concentrated liquids has been replaced by a safer and far superior product for feeding hypercaloric milk

**Tabel 22.1** Hypercaloric feedings with formula/human milk mixture of formula

| Milk at 100 kilocalories | mL | Protein (g) | Fat (g) | CHO (g) | Ca (mg) | P (mg) |
|---|---|---|---|---|---|---|
| PTHM + SHMF + SSC30 to 27 kcal/ounce | 111 | 3 | 6 | 9 | 178 | 100 |
| PTHM + SHMF + SSC30 to 28 kcal/ounce | 106 | 3 | 6.23 | 8.5 | 179 | 100 |
| SSC 30 | 100 | 3 | 6.61 | 7.7 | 180 | 100 |

PTHM, preterm human milk.
SHMF, Similac Human Milk Fortifier (Abbott Nutritionals, Columbus, OH).
SSC30, Similac Special Care 30.

to formula-fed VLBW infants (Table 22.1). These mixtures can provide 27 and 28 kilocalories/ounce.

Therefore the VLBW infant can receive the same quantity of protein as with standard preterm formulas but with less volume. The calories from fat are increased and carbohydrate calories are lower versus standard preterm formula. The osmolarity at 30 cal/ounce is 325 mOsm versus preterm formula at 280. This liquid enables the clinician to feed hypercalorically and maintain protein intake for both formula-fed fluid-restricted VLBW infants and for those infants receiving mother's milk who also require fluid restriction.

Finally, there is now a human milk fortifier prepared from human donor milk which allows the formulation of 26–30 kilocalorie per ounce human milk. This can also be added to mother's milk or donor human milk to provide exclusive human milk and take advantage of human milk feedings even in VLBW infants requiring fluid restriction (Table 22.2).

**Table 22.2**  Hypercaloric human milk feeding for very low birthweight infants (≤ 1500 g BW)

|  | Fortifier | | | |
| --- | --- | --- | --- | --- |
|  | Prolact +4 | +6 | +8 | +10 |
| *Per 100 ml* | | | | |
| OMM or BBM | 80/20 | 70/30 | 60/40 | 50/50 |
| Energy | 83 | 91 | 98 | 104 |
| Protein (g) | 2.4 | 2.8 | 3.3 | 3.8 |
| OSM | <335 | 337 | 347 | 349 |
| *Per 120 kcal/kg/d* | | | | |
| Protein | 3.5 | 3.7 | 4.0 | 4.3 |
| Volume | 145 | 132 | 122 | 115 |
| Ca | 186 | 169 | 156 | 177 |
| P | 102 | 92 | 85 | 99 |

All of these strategies collectively provide enough energy with adequate protein for growth with hypercaloric feedings in fluid-restricted infants. Figure 22.1 illustrates these strategies depending on the degree of fluid restriction. There may be a role for these 26–30 kcal/ounce options in VLBW infants who are not fluid-restricted. These are infants with severe postnatal growth failure despite receiving adequate volumes of preterm formula or fortified human milk. Particularly if the growth failure includes head circumference below the 10th percentile (symmetric growth failure) a short (7–10 day) trial of full-volume feeding of these milks will provide both increased intake of protein and energy. The protein/energy ratio will be low with the formula mixture.

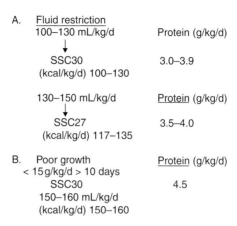

Figure 22.1 Hypercaloric feedings with formula

# Growth in the neonatal intensive care unit influences neurodevelopmental and growth outcomes

A recent multicenter cohort study from the original NICHD growth observation study included a large number of infants with birthweights from 501 to 1000 g to determine the effect of growth rates during hospitalization on neurodevelopment. These infants were stratified by 100 g birthweight increments and divided into quartiles based on in-hospital growth velocity rates. As the rate of weight gain increased between quartile 1 and quartile 4, from 12.0 to 21.2 g/kg/d, the incidence of cerebral palsy, Bayley II Mental Developmental Index (MDI) scores of less than 70, Psychomotor Developmental Index scores of less than 70, abnormal neurologic examination findings, neurodevelopmental impairment including blindness and deafness, and need for rehospitalization fell significantly at 18 to 22 months corrected age. Similar findings were observed as rate of head circumference growth increased from 0.67 to 1.12 cm/week from quartile 1 to quartile 4 respectively. Head circumference gain of more than 0.9 cm/week was associated with better neurodevelopmental and growth outcomes.

In addition, higher in-hospital growth rates were associated with a decreased likelihood of anthropometric measurements below the 10th percentile at 18 months corrected age. The influence of growth velocity remained after controlling for

Better neurodevelopmental and growth
outcomes ELBW

Weight gain ≥ 18 g/kg/d
HC > 0.9 cm/week

If those rates falter, the infant's diet should
be reviewed and modified to achieve the
target growth parameters.

Ehrenkranz et al. Peds April 2006

**Figure 23.1  Growth in NICU and neurodevelopment.**

variables known at birth or identified during the infants'
neonatal intensive care unit hospitalizations which could
affect outcomes.

This study emphasizes the importance of closely
monitoring the rate of in-hospital growth once birthweight
has been regained. If rates of growth are faltering, the infant's
diet should be reviewed and modifications can be made
to achieve the target growth parameters of weight gain
greater than or equal to 18 g/kg/d and head circumference
growth of > 0.9 cm/week from return to birthweight through to
discharge (Figure 23.1).

## SUGGESTED READING

Ehrenkranz RA, Dusick AM, Vohr BR, Wright LL, Wrage LA,
Poole WK. Growth in the neonatal intensive care unit
influences neurodevelopmental and growth outcomes of
extremely low birth weight infants. *Pediatrics* 2006; **117**:
1253–1261.

# Chapter 24

# Nutritional assessment

An in-depth nutritional assessment requires dietary, anthropometric, biochemical, and clinical data. However, the taking of anthropometric and biochemical measurements is difficult; therefore, nutritional assessment in neonates receiving intensive care treatment is frequently confined to detecting fluctuations in weight gain and in caloric intake. Nonetheless, it is necessary for the clinician to be able to assess the neonate's nutritional status because of the potentially serious sequelae of malnutrition on multiple organ systems and the importance of growth (especially brain growth) to developmental outcome. The provision of energy and nutrients at levels to support growth and development is the goal of nutrition support for VLBW infants.

Nutritional assessment includes considering the length of gestation and adequacy of intrauterine growth as well as nutrient tolerance. Static assessment (current balance between intake and output) as well as a dynamic assessment (evaluation of infant's growth over time or growth velocity) of each infant are both important. Also, the nonnutritional factors such as disease state, morbidities, and medications must be considered.

## Body weight

Weight gain is the most frequently used anthropometric measure. It is important to use the same scale, obtain weight measurements at the same time each day to avoid diurnal variations, and indicate any equipment being weighed (especially arm boards and dressings); if equipment is not recorded, changes in weight may be spurious. In preterm infants, weight gain should be expressed on a gram per kilogram per day basis.

When assessing weight, there are several issues to consider. Body weight comprises the total mass of the infant's lean tissue, fat, and extracellular fluid compartments. In the first week of life, all newborns lose weight as a result of loss or contraction of extracellular fluid, free water and low intake; however, most VLBW infants may be also calorie- and fluid-restricted during that period as a result of illness or nutritional practices. Therefore, it may be difficult to separate changes in growth measurements caused by diuresis from those caused by poor protein–calorie intake. Weight gain does not necessarily reflect growth, which is a deposition of new tissue of normal composition; weight increase may reflect excessive fat deposition or water retention, neither of which is truly growth. Weight gain or loss reflects changes in body composition.

Earlier studies reported postnatal weight loss of up to 20% of total body weight in ELBW infants. This included loss of lean tissue in the absence of adequate energy and nutrients. Recently, initial postnatal weight loss of ≤ 10% of total body

**Table 24.1** Postnatal weight loss, subsequent gain, and growth velocities from selected references

|  | Weight Loss (% of BW) | Birth Weight Regained (days) | Weight (g/kg/d) | Length (cm/week) | Head Circumference (cm/week) |
|---|---|---|---|---|---|
| Shaffer | 10–20 | 13–15 | 14.8 |  |  |
| Wright | 10–20 | 13–15 | 20.8 | 0.90 | 0.72 |
| Ehrenkranz | 7–10 | 11–17 | 15.0 | 0.98 | 0.92 |
| Christensen | 0–5 | 0–9 | 15.0 |  |  |

*Note*: All listed references reported initial weight loss and days to regain birth greater in smaller, more immature infants, with the exception of Christensen. From LJ Mayer-Mileur. Anthropometric and laboratory assessment of very low birthweight infants: the most helpful measurements and why. *Semin Perinatol* 2007; 31 (2).

weight has been observed with changes in fluid management with early TPN and MEN in ELBW infants. Table 24.1 demonstrates weight-related data from various references between 1987 and 2006.

## Length

Length measurements are the most inaccurate anthropometric measurement. Accurate technique is important in performing length measurements to detect small changes. Two trained individuals are needed to measure the infant on a measuring board containing a stationary head board, a moveable foot board, and a built-in tape measure. Skeletal growth is often spared relative to weight in mildly malnourished infants; therefore, initially, linear grow is often slow or stops. Serial length measures obtained weekly are helpful in assessing nutritional status when plotted over time; length measures are especially useful in infants with BPD, whose weight fluctuates greatly. A gain in length of 1 cm per week is expected.

## Head circumference

Increase in head circumference (HC), the measurement of the largest occipitofrontal circumference, correlates well with cellular growth of the brain and with brain weight as well. Therefore, measuring HC is really a surrogate for monitoring brain growth. During acute illness the velocity of head growth for the sick preterm infant is less than that of the normal fetus. During recovery, head growth parallels that of normal fetal growth and subsequently rapid "catch-up" growth in HC may occur. Normal brain growth may not occur until the acute illness has resolved, despite high energy intake. Those preterm infants calorically deprived for the longest periods showed slower growth rates and longer duration of catch-up growth. The longer these infants remain with suboptimal head size, the greater is their developmental risk. Head growth correlates well with overall growth during fetal development, infancy and early childhood. It also correlates well with developmental achievement in VLBW infants.

HC is usually measured once a week using a paper tape; a new tape should be used for each infant. A goal of about 0.9 cm per week is to be expected. If hydrocephalus is a concern, more frequent measures are warranted. The initial HC may differ from subsequent measurements because of molding of the head. Measuring HC may be difficult as a result of interfering equipment such as intravenous lines on the scalp.

Serial weight, length, and HC measurements should be placed on an appropriate growth chart. Daily weights may be plotted on the Hall or Fenton growth chart or weekly on the Benda and Babson growth chart, or the Ehrenkranz NICHD growth observation curve. A summary of postnatal growth curves spanning 1948 to 2005 is shown in Table 24.2.

Skin-fold measures of several sites have been used to estimate body fat stores and the percent body fat in children and adults. These determinations use a variety of formulas that are based on the assumption that the percent of TBW and fat distribution remains constant. However, in the neonate, these assumptions are not valid because percent body water decreases with increasing gestational age and postnatal age and fat increases with increasing gestational age.

The biochemical assessment of nutritional status may be more specific than anthropometric measures. Biochemical assessment may be useful when used in combination with anthropometric indices for nutritional assessment of the sick neonate. Many routine tests may signal nutrition-related problems. For example, an elevated alkaline phosphatase level (>1000 IU) and a low serum phosphorus (<4 mg/dL) may occur during the active phase of osteopenia of prematurity. This combination of biochemical findings indicates the need to obtain diagnostic X-ray studies. However, abnormal alkaline phosphatase levels may occur as a result of hepatic dysfunction. Heat fractionation of the isoenzyme is suggested to determine its origin. As osteopenia improves,

SINGLETON HOSPITAL
STAFF LIBRARY

**Table 24.2.** Summary of select postnatal growth charts for VLBW infants

| Author | Birth years | N | Exclusions | GA and/or Birth weight | Anthropometric measurements | Growth period |
|---|---|---|---|---|---|---|
| Danics | 1948 | 100 | major congenital anomalies | 1000–2500 g | daily weight | 50 days |
| Shaffer | 1984–1985 | 385 | major congenital anomalies | 500–2500 g | daily weight | 40 days |
| Wright | 1987–1991 | 205 | major congenital anomalies; NEC | 501–1500 g | daily weight, weekly length and OFC | 105 days |
| Ehrenkranz | 1994–1995 | 1660 | major congenital anomalies | 501–1500 g | daily weight, weekly length, OFC, & midarm circumference | 120 days |
| Christensen | 2003–2005 | 1813 | none | 23 to 42 wks 400 to 2600 g | daily weight | 100 days |
| IHDP | 1985 | 212 | major congenital anomalies | 501 to 1500 g | weight, length, & OFC: monthly to 6 months; every 2 months from 6 to 12 months; every 3 months from 12 to 36 months | 32 wks–36 mo |

From LJ Meyer-Mileur. Anthropometric and laboratory assessment of very low birthweight infants: the most helpful measurements and why. *Semin Perinatol* 2007; 31 (2).

the serum phosphorus levels normalize, whereas the alkaline phosphatase continues to be elevated during the radiographic healing. Elevated alkaline phosphatase levels generally precede radiologic changes by two to four weeks.

Albumin is a serum protein commonly measured in routine laboratory tests. While it has limited value for nutritional assessment, a low albumin may serve as an indicator of inadequate energy and protein intake. The average serum albumin concentration in infants less than 37 weeks gestation ranges from 2.0 to 2.7 g/dL. This relative hypoalbuminemia of the preterm infant appears to be as a result of a more rapid turnover of a small plasma pool as opposed to a decreased rate of albumin synthesis; the half-life of albumin is approximately 7.5 days in the preterm infant as compared with 14.8 days in adults. Despite the relatively rapid turnover, serum albumin concentration changes slowly in response to nutrition rehabilitation.

Therefore to quickly assess response to nutrition support, a serum protein with a shorter half-life is necessary. Transthyretin (prealbumin), with a half-life of approximately two days in adults, has been shown to be a suitable marker for evaluation of nutritional status in VLBW infants. Transthyretin increases with gestational age as well as with protein and energy intake. The direction of change in serial tests may be more useful than striving for absolute values. Transthyretin is not a very sensitive indicator overall and most clinicians rely on growth velocity and growth curves to assess response to nutrition support.

The VLBW infant is subject to various metabolic, renal, respiratory, and gastrointestinal abnormalities, and therefore close monitoring of blood gases, serum electrolytes, calcium, phosphorus, glucose, BUN, and creatinine are standard and necessary.

Ongoing nutritional assessment includes careful calculation of dietary intake relative to estimated requirements, determination of fluid balance and hydration status, and tolerance to feeding method. In combination with anthropometric, clinical, and biochemical data, adjustments in intake or method of nutrient delivery can be made to achieve effective nutritional support.

### SUGGESTED READING

Anderson D. Nutritional assessment and therapeutic interventions for preterm infant. *Clin Perinatol* 2002; **29**:313–326.

Christensen RD, Henry E, Kiehn TI, et al. Pattern of daily weights among low birth weight neonates in the neonatal intensive care unit: data from multihospital health-care system. *J Perinatol* 2006; **26**:37–43.

Ehrenkranz RA, Tounes N, Lemons JA, et al. Longitudinal growth of hospitalized very low birth weight infants. *Pediatrics* 1999; **104**:280–289.

Fenton T. A new growth chart for preterm babies: Babson and Benda's chart updated with recent data and a new format. *BMC Pediatr* 2003; **3**:13–16.

Moyer-Mileur LJ, Brunstetter VL, McNaught T, et al. Physical activity program increases bone mineralization and growth in preterm very low birth weight infants. *Pediatrics* 2000; **106**:1088–1092.

Shaffer SG, Quimiro CL, Anderson JV, et al. Postnatal weight changes in very low birth weight infants. *Pediatrics* 1987; **70**:702–705.

Wright K, Dawson JP, Fallis D, et al. New postnatal growth grids for very low birth weight infants. *Pediatrics* 1993; **91**:922–926.

# Chapter 25

# Post-discharge strategies

Although considerable attention has been directed toward improving the nutrition of hospitalized VLBW infants with nutrient-enriched formulas and multinutrient fortifiers for human milk, only recently has attention been paid to nutrition support of such infants after hospital discharge. The first postnatal year provides an important opportunity for human somatic and brain growth to compensate for earlier deprivation (see Fig. 25.1). It is probable that VLBW infants have special nutrient requirements in the post-discharge period. In more biologic terms, it is reasonable to ask whether this period is also critical for later health and development, as it is common for human milk fortifiers to be stopped or term formulas to be substituted for preterm formulas at hospital discharge. Available data suggest that preterm infants are in a state of suboptimal nutrition at the time of discharge and are frequently below the tenth percentile on the growth curve, which may be referred to as extrauterine growth restriction. These VLBW infants have also accumulated significant nutrient deficits by the time of discharge. Improving these deficits is beneficial both in the short term and, potentially, for longer-term health and development.

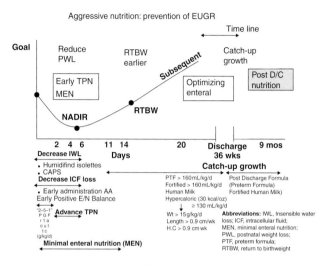

Figure 25.1  Aggressive nutrition: prevention of EUGR. Adamkin DH. Feeding the preterm infant. In: J Bhatia, ed. *Perinatal Nutrition Optimizing Infant Health and Development.* New York, NY: Marcel Dekker; 2004: 165–190. Reproduced with permission.

Nutrient-enriched formula for preterm infants after hospital discharge (post-discharge formula: PDF) is generally intermediate in composition between preterm and term formulas. Table 25.1 shows the nutrient concentrations provided by various diets fed at 200 mL/kg/d after discharge. Compared with term formula (TF), PDF contains an increased amount of protein with sufficient additional energy 22 kcal/ounce to permit utilization. PDF contains extra calcium, phosphorus, and zinc, all of which are necessary to promote linear growth.

**Table 25.1** Macronutrients supplied by commonly used formulas for preterm infants at the time of discharge, assuming an intake of 200 mL/kg/day

| | Target | Human milk | Similac[a] Advance w/Fe 20 kcal/oz | Enfamil Lipil[b] w/Fe 20 kcal/oz | Similac[a] Neosure Advance 22 kcal/oz | Enfacare[b] Lipil 22 kcal/oz |
|---|---|---|---|---|---|---|
| Calories/kg | 120–130 | 138 | 136 | 136 | 150 | 148 |
| Protein g/kg | 2.5–3.5 | 2.0 | 2.8 | 2.8 | 4.2 | 4.2 |
| Fat g/kg | 6.0–8.0 | 7.8 | 7.2 | 7.2 | 8.2 | 7.8 |
| CHO g/kg | 10–14 | 13.2 | 14.6 | 14.6 | 15.4 | 15.8 |
| Vitamin A IU/kg | 1000 | 780 | 406 | 406 | 686 | 666 |
| Vitamin D IU | 200–400 | 4 | 80 | 80 | 104 | 118 |
| Vitamin E IU/kg | 6–12 | 2.0 | 4.0 | 2.6 | 5.4 | 6.0 |
| Ca mg/kg | 150–175 | 50 | 106 | 106 | 156 | 178 |
| P mg/kg | 90–105 | 26 | 56 | 72 | 92 | 98 |
| Fe mg/kg | 2–4 | 0.2 | 2.4 | 2.4 | 2.6 | 2.6 |

Adapted form American Academy of Pediatrics: *Pediatric Nutrition Handbook*, 5th ed. 2004, Appendices A and E.

[a] From Abbott Nutritionals Products.

[b] From Mead Johnson Nutritionals.

Adapted from Greer FR, Post discharge nutrition: what does the evidence support? *Semin Perinatol* 2007; 31 (2).

With permission.

Additional vitamins and trace elements are included to support the projected increased growth. Table 25.2 shows growth velocity for preterm infants from term to 24 months. A pilot study of 32 preterm infants performed 15 years ago was the first

**Table 25.2** Growth velocity of preterm infants from term to 24 months (range includes ± 1SD)

| Age from term (months) | Weight (g/day) | Length (cm/month) | Head circumference (cm/month) |
|---|---|---|---|
| 1 | 26–40 | 3.0–4.5 | 1.6–2.5 |
| 4 | 15–25 | 2.3–3.6 | 0.8–1.4 |
| 8 | 12–17 | 1.0–2.0 | 0.3–0.8 |
| 12 | 9–12 | 0.8–15 | 0.2–0.4 |
| 18 | 4–10 | 0.7–1.3 | 0.1–04 |

From Theriot L. Routine nutrition care during follow up. In: S Groh-Wargo, M Thompson and JH Cox, eds. *Nutrition Care for High Risk Newborns.* Chicago, IL: Precept Press; 2000: 570. With permission.

to demonstrate that infants randomized to receive the PDF up to nine months post-term showed significantly greater weight and length gains and had higher bone mineral content in the distal radius than infants who received a standard term formula.

Three subsequent studies provide insight into the role of PDF, suggesting that benefits may be related to birthweight, gender and a specific postconceptual age when supplemental nutrients can promote catch-up and subsequent growth. Two of the reports also raise the possibility that post-discharge nutrition may benefit long-term development.

A total of 284 preterm infants in a United Kingdom multicenter study received either TF or PDF for the first 9 months post-term. At 9 months post-term, PDF-fed infants were significantly heavier (mean difference, 370 g) and longer (1.1 cm) than TF-fed infants; only the length difference persisted to 18 months post-term or nine months after discontinuation of the PDF. Differences between diet groups were significantly greater in boys, who had a length advantage of 1.5 cm at 18 months if they received PDF. There was no evidence that the PDF had promoted fat accretion, as mean weight percentile was still below the 50th percentile, and skin-fold thicknesses were not increased. Therefore the increased growth was consistent with lean mass. Head circumference and developmental outcome at nine or 18 months did not differ significantly between groups, although PDF-fed infants had a 2.8-point advantage (0.25 SD) in Bayley MDI Score (the study was powered to detect a larger [0.30 SD] difference)

The Carver USA multicenter study reported improved growth in preterm infants fed a PDF after hospital discharge up to 12 months corrected age, with the significant differences in weight, length, or head circumference most marked for smaller infants (birthweight < 1250 g) and again male infants. The differences in growth produced by PDF occurred early and then were sustained over time, suggesting that the most rapid catch-up with respect to using PDF occurred soon after discharge between 40 and 48 weeks. Infants with the lowest birthweights, less than 1250 g, also experienced enhanced growth in head circumference.

The third study examined the use of preterm formula (PTF 24 kcal/ounce) after discharge in 129 preterm infants randomly assigned to one of three dietary regimens until six months post-term: TF, PTF, or PTF until term followed by TF to six months. Males fed PTF after discharge showed significantly greater weight and length gain and larger head circumference by six months post-term than those fed TF throughout the study period. Infants fed PTF consumed an average 180 mL/kg, resulting in a protein intake of approximately 4 g/kg per day. Those fed TF increased consumption to about 220 mL/kg per day, but their protein intake did not match that of the PTF group. At 18 months post-term, boys previously fed PTF were on average 1 kg heavier, 1 cm longer and had 1 cm greater head circumference than those fed TF. Body composition measurements using dual X-ray absorptiometry suggested that the additional weight gain was composed predominantly of lean tissue rather than fat. There were no significant differences in neurodevelopment measured using the Bayley Scales of Infant Development at 18 months. PTF post-discharge is not a routinely used strategy for VLBW infants. However, it might be considered for those infants with symmetric growth failure (HC and weight <10th percentile) at discharge to take advantage of the critical growth epoch between 40 and 48 weeks. The enhanced protein and energy might allow for maximal catch-up during this "window of opportunity." After the two months these infants should be placed back on the PDF.

Randomized studies demonstrated that the use of either PTF or PDF after discharge in preterm infants results in improved growth, with differences in weight and length persisting beyond the period of intervention. Such findings suggest that nutrition during the post-discharge period may have longer-term effects on growth trajectory. Evidence from three randomized trials suggests that the effect of a nutrient-enriched post-discharge diet is greatest in boys, possibly reflecting their higher growth rates and protein requirements.

Several nonrandomized controlled trials have shown that breastfed infants do not grow as well as their formula-fed counterparts after discharge. Options include replacing some breast feeds with nutrient-enriched formula feed or fortifying expressed breast milk. Recent information from the post-discharge feeding study group mixed one half of the human milk fed each day to human milk-fed ($\geq 80\%$ feeding per day) preterm infants with four packets of a powdered multinutrient human milk fortifier for 12 weeks after discharge.

This strategy did not influence human milk feeding when intensive lactation support was provided. Infants in the intervention group were longer during the study period and those born $\leq 1250$ g had larger head circumferences.

## PRACTICAL TIPS for post-discharge

Discharge preterm infants EGA $\leq 34$ weeks or birthweight < 1800 g on post-discharge formula

Follow anthropometrics carefully post-discharge and maintain the PDF strategy 9–12 months corrected age especially for VLBW infants

VLBW infants discharged feeding human milk require an individualized approach based on anthropometrics and whether or not there is evidence of osteopenia of prematurity developing pre- or post-discharge

Human-milk-fed babies with growth failure or evidence of osteopenia may receive fortification by mixing feedings with the post-discharge milk or fortification strategies alluded to in the human milk and hypercaloric sections

Growth post-discharge should be monitored with the CDC, NCHS Growth Curves and not the IHDP Curves

## SUGGESTED READING

Adamkin DH. Postdischarge nutritional therapy. *J Perinatol* 2006; **26**(suppl 1):S27–S30.

American Academy of Pediatrics, Committee on Nutrition. Nutritional needs of preterm infants. In: RE Kleinman, ed. *Pediatric Nutrition Handbook*. 5th ed. Elk Grove Village, IL: American Academy of Pediatrics; 2004: 23–54.

Carver J. Nutrition for preterm infants after hospital discharge. *Adv Pediatr* 2005; **5 2**:23–47.

Carver JD, Wu PYK, Hall RT, et al. Growth of preterm infants fed nutrient-enriched or term formula after hospital discharge. *Pediatrics* 2001; **107**:683.

Cooke RJ, Embleton ND, Giffin IJ, Wells JC, McCormick KP. Feeding preterm infants after hospital discharge: growth and development at 18 months of age. *Pediatr Res* 2001; **49**:719.

Embleton NE, Pang N, Cooke RJ. Postnatal malnutrition and growth retardation: an inevitable consequence of current recommendations in preterm infants? *Pediatrics* 2001; **107**:270–273.

Ernst KD, Radmacher PG, Rafail ST, et al. Postnatal
   malnutrition of extremely low birth-weight infants with
   catch-up growth postdischarge. *J Perinatol* 2003; **23**:447–482.
O'Connor DL, Khan S, Welshuhn K, et al. Growth and nutrient
   intakes of human milk-fed preterm infants provided
   with extra energy and nutrients after hospital discharge.
   *Pediatrics* 2008; **121** (4).

# Chapter 26

# Nutritional management of preterm infants with short bowel syndrome

## Introduction

The Short Bowel Syndrome (SBS) is the loss of intestinal length and absorptive surface area due to surgical resection. The loss of this mucosal absorptive surface area results in malabsorption and rapid transit potentiating malnutrition, recurrent dehydration, and electrolyte abnormalities. The most common cause of SBS in preterm infants is necrotizing enterocolitis with extensive resection. Other causes include resection following congenital malformations such as midgut volvulus from malrotation, intestinal atresias, and gastroschisis. VLBW infants with SBS require total parenteral nutrition (TPN) to provide the essential nutrients to sustain life and promote growth. The remaining bowel may be insufficient in length and function to utilize enteral nutrition. More than 80% of infants and children survive after extensive small bowel resection in the neonatal period. Prognosis is related to adjusted intestinal length, the presence of an ileocecal valve, colon preservation and occurrence of cholestasis. Most of the deaths in patients with SBS are caused by liver failure or sepsis and occur during the first year of life. The time for which the infant is dependent on TPN is significantly influenced by the length of residual intestine and the absence of an ileocecal valve. The goal in the nutritional management of these infants is to gradually advance enteral nutrient delivery while the residual bowel adapts, and simultaneously weaning and discontinuing TPN while avoiding life-threatening liver disease. Ultimately the goal is for the infant to achieve normal growth and development by consuming an oral diet.

The clinical presentation of infants with SBS varies widely and is dependent on the age of the infant at the time of intestinal resection, the length of remaining bowel, the area of the bowel resected and the presence or absence of the ileocecal valve and colon. A full-term infant is born with approximately 200–300 cm of small bowel. The bowel doubles in length during the third trimester and it is thought that an infant born prematurely has a greater potential for the bowel to grow linearly than a term infant. The bowel continues to lengthen for the first few years of life and the rate of lengthening levels off at about 3 to 4 years of age. Therefore, the younger the infant or child is the more opportunity the bowel will have to increase in length and the more likely bowel adaptation will occur. The length of bowel remaining is also indicative of the ability of the infant to be weaned from parenteral nutrition. However, it is also dependent on the functionality of the remaining bowel. Removal of the jejunum may result in malabsorption of macronutrients (nitrogen, fat, and carbohydrate) as well as nutritional deficiencies such as iron, calcium, and magnesium. Resection of the ileum may result in vitamin B12 deficiency and thus serum levels must be monitored and supplemented accordingly. The ileum releases hormones responsible for regulating transit time. The absence of the ileum can potentially lead to diarrhea. Steatorrhea may also result from an inadequate bile salt pool resulting in fat-soluble vitamin and zinc deficiency. Preservation of the ileum improves the prognosis of bowel adaptation. The ileum can compensate for the functions lost by the removal of the jejunum. In the absence of the ileocecal valve bacteria from the colon reflux into the small intestine and cause bacterial overgrowth resulting in diarrhea and ultimately preventing the advancement of enteral feeds. The emptying of the small intestinal contents into the colon is not regulated in the absence of the ileocecal valve, thus resulting in further malabsorption from lack of time for adequate absorption of nutrients. The loss of the colon may result in severe dehydration from diarrhea due to inadequate fluid and electrolyte absorption as well as hyponatremia, hypokalemia, and hypomagnesemia. Therefore, knowledge of the remaining bowel is critical to the nutritional management of an infant with SBS.

## Intestinal adaptation

Hypertrophy and hyperplasia of the residual bowel begins within 48 hours of partial bowel resection and is complete within 3-6 months. Adaptation continues at a very slow rate and may take several years. The intestine continues to adapt by increasing the number of enterocytes per villus, its rate of proliferation, and villus height. The bowel slowly dilates to increase the surface area and delays transit time to further maximize nutrient absorption. However, this dilatation

may not be advantageous as it can lead to small bowel
bacterial overgrowth and potentially bacterial translocation,
deconjugation of bile acids and D-lactic acidemia. The ability
of the small intestine to adapt depends largely on exposure to
enteral nutrients. Enteral nutrients also promote the release
of hormones, which slow transit time, and increase villus
height and fluid absorption. Therefore, infants who are unable
to tolerate even minimal continuous feedings may suffer
from mucosal atrophy. However, once enteral nutrients are
reintroduced, mucosal hypertrophy should begin.

## Nutrition therapy

In a retrospective review Javid et al. (2005 a,b) reported that
TPN-dependent infants who transitioned to full enteral
nutrition achieved normalization of hyperbilirubinemia
within 4 months of discontinuation of TPN. They stated that
these findings support aggressive weaning of TPN to enteral
nutrition in infants with short bowel syndrome. Attempt to
obtain optimal growth while avoiding over-feeding. Special
attention on maintaining weight/length between the 25th and
75th percentile is needed. Careful monitoring of electrolytes
calcium, phosphorus, magnesium, and zinc is necessary
as their stomal losses may be excessive. In addition, trace
metals such as zinc, selenium, copper, and manganese
must be monitored every three months so adjustments in
the parenteral nutrition can be made in a timely manner.
Meticulous care of the central line is required to prevent
sepsis. When enteral nutrition is successfully advanced, TPN

may begin to be weaned. Cycling of the TPN for 2–4 hours daily may be attempted if the infant is able to maintain blood glucose levels. Enteral nutrition should be initiated post-resection once ileus has resolved. As enteral calories are increased parenteral calories are simultaneously decreased. It is important to note that enteral calorie needs will be ≥ 10% higher than parenteral calories due to metabolism and variable amounts of malabsorption. There is no specific formula that is recommended for infants with SBS. Breast milk has many well-known advantages and is an excellent source of growth factors but may not be optimally absorbed. The literature reports that protein is better tolerated than other nutrients. Intact proteins stimulate mucosal hyperplasia more than protein hydrolysates. However, in light of the reduced absorptive surface area partially hydrolyzed formulas may be better tolerated and are most commonly utilized. In the presence of heme-positive stools an amino acid-based formula should be considered. The benefits of an amino acid-based formula over a protein hydrolysate-based formula are unclear. Infants with SBS are predisposed to intestinal mucosal barrier breakdown, bowel dilatation, and bacterial overgrowth, and are at increased risk for developing protein allergies. Infant formulas containing amino acids as the protein source are Elecare and Neocate. Elecare contains 33% and Neocate contains 5% of fat calories as medium-chain triglyceride (MCT). Elecare may be preferable in an infant with SBS, severe protein allergy and fat malabsorption. A disadvantage of amino acid-based formulas is their higher osmolality, which can cause osmotic diarrhea and result in the inability to advance in volume and/or caloric concentration. Carbohydrate content of the formula should ideally be no more than 40% of calories to prevent an excessive osmotic load to the gut and to avoid bacterial overgrowth. Long-chain triglycerides (LCT) stimulate intestinal adaptation after intestinal resection. Infants with SBS may experience fat malabsorption due to bile salt malabsorption, which leads to decreased micelle formation and fat digestion. Infants with bile acid or pancreatic insufficiency may therefore tolerate MCT better than LCT as MCT does not require micelle formation. However, MCT also increases the osmotic load in the intestine and provides fewer calories than LCT. Therefore, an infant formula containing both MCT and LCT is recommended for improved energy and fat absorption.

Providing continuous enteral nutrition allows for constant saturation of intestinal transporters, thus using the full extent of the remaining absorptive surface area. Mucosal hyperplasia is stimulated through direct contact with epithelial cells; stimulation of gastric, biliary, and pancreatic secretions; and enhanced production of trophic hormones. Bolus feedings are another method of providing enteral nutrition in older children, but are poorly tolerated in preterm infants with SBS. Enteral feedings should be advanced slowly as clinically tolerated. One way to assess tolerance is to assess fecal reducing substances and fecal pH. Reducing substances should be < 1% and stool pH should be > 5.5. Carbohydrate malabsorption is identified if fecal reducing substances are > 1 % and fecal pH is < 5.5. Another way to assess tolerance is to monitor ostomy output, with a goal 40–50 mL/kg/day.

Feeding aversion is a very common occurrence among this population as a result of lack of introduction of oral feedings, lack of hunger/satiety response, orally invasive procedures such as mechanical ventilation and administration of unpleasant-tasting medications. It is critical to initiate and maintain minimal oral feeding and/or oral stimulation therapy with speech and/or occupational therapists as early as possible. As little as 5 mL of formula given orally daily will improve outcome.

## Soluble fiber

Protracted diarrhea prevents the advancement of enteral feedings and prolongs dependence on PN. Clinical practice has included the addition of fiber to EN to reduce stool and/or ostomy output. Sources of fiber include pectin, green beans, and guar gum. Soluble fiber is fermented in the colon to produce short-chain fatty acids (SCFA) that provide fuel to colonocytes, stimulate epithelial cell proliferation and exert a trophic effect on the colonic mucosa. SCFA stimulate sodium transport in the colon and thus water absorption. Pectin is a type of soluble fiber that is an amylase-resistant polysaccharide found in the cell wall of many fruits and vegetables. Pectin may decrease gastrointestinal transit time and improved nitrogen absorption, with no adverse effect on electrolyte balance or glucose absorption. Certo liquid pectin (1–3% or 1–3 mL pectin/100 mL formula) is currently recommended. Higher doses are generally avoided because of the hyperosmotic effect resulting in more diarrhea.

## Lengthening procedures

Surgical bowel-lengthening procedures are used in infants with SBS who fail to tolerate advancement of enteral nutrition. Such surgeries facilitate bowel adaptation by increasing the surface area of the bowel, prolong transit time and thus enhance absorption. Infants with dilated bowel segments may qualify for either a serial transverse enteroplasty (STEP) as described by Javid et al. (2005 a,b) or an intestinal lengthening and tapering (LILT) described by Bianchi in 1997 and DiBaise et al. in 2004. They do not recommend the LILT procedure be performed in patients with severe liver disease. These procedures may be beneficial when ineffective peristalsis and bacterial overgrowth develop following intestinal dilatation with the goal of optimizing bowel adaptation and absorption over time.

## Drug therapy

Pharmacologic therapy has been utilized to manage infants with SBS and includes the use of antimotility agents, antisecretory drugs, and antimicrobials. Loperamide is often used to slow transit rate and increase water and nutrient absorption. It acts directly on the intestinal muscles to inhibit peristalsis. A typical dose of 0.8 mg/kg/d to a maximum of 24 mg/d in the liquid form is recommended but should not be used in infants with refractory small bowel bacterial overgrowth. Cholestyramine may be useful in reducing secretory diarrhea in patients with ileal resection and loose, watery stools.

However, in patients with fat malabsorption due to bile salt insufficiency, cholestyramine may actually worsen diarrhea and increase the risk of deficiency of fat-soluble vitamins. Ursodial is a hydrophilic bile acid used to prevent or treat TPNAC. It improves bile acid flow and displaces toxic acids. It reduces signs and symptoms of cholestasis but does not prevent disease progression. Ursodial may cause diarrhea. Small bowel bacterial overgrowth is a common complication in infants with SBS especially in the absence of the ileocecal valve, poor motility of a dilated small bowel segment or in the presence of a restrictive anastomosis. Small bowel bacterial overgrowth may increase the risk of intestinal bacterial translocation and complicate the advancement and tolerance of enteral feeding. It predisposes infants to sepsis. Bacterial overgrowth results in inflammation of the mucosal surface area and impairs bowel adaptation and results in diarrhea and weight loss. Ching et al. (2007) discuss the use of short courses of oral antimicrobials to reduce bacterial overgrowth. Typically they are given for a 1 week period per month. In order to prevent the development of resistance various agents may be rotated .

## Conclusion

Infants with SBS are unique and their management is challenging. Long-term TPN remains a very effective therapy to support these patients and provide them with an opportunity to grow and develop as their bowel adapts. The goal in infants with SBS requiring long-term TPN is to transition to full enteral nutrition or oral diet while avoiding

life-threatening liver failure. Optimum nutrition support
should provide adequate hydration, calories, and nutrients to
ensure survival of the infant, proper growth, and development.
The management of these infants requires comprehensive
care from a multidisciplinary team involving neonatologists,
pediatric surgeons, gastroenterologists, dietitians, specialized
nurses, social workers, occupational therapists, and speech
therapists. Infants who develop complications associated
with long-term dependency on TPN may be candidates
for combined small bowel–liver or isolated intestinal
transplantation.

**PRACTICAL TIPS for managing nutrition in short bowel syndrome**

1. Monitor ostomy output with a goal of 40–50 mL/kg/day;
   if there is significant increase in output or electrolyte
   abnormalities advancement of feeding schedule should
   be reevaluated

2. Gradual introduction of enteral feedings by
   continuous drip followed by advancement of enteral
   feeds

3. Early referral to an experienced pediatric intestinal
   transplant center/pediatric gastrointestinal center for
   further assessment is recommended in infants with poor
   prognosis or if TPN for > 3 months

4. Consider medications, probiotics, limiting I.V. lipid to 1
   g/kg/day, utilization of an omega–3 I.V. lipid to prevent
   or reverse hepatic injury

5. Monitor growth parameters

6. Monitor trace elements during long-term delivery of TPN such as zinc, selenium, copper, manganese, and chromium once infant has developed liver cholestasis (direct bilirubin > 2 mg/dL) or received TPN for > 3 months

7. Measure triene/tetraene ratio to assess essential fatty acid deficiency

8. Monitor carnitine ratio and supplement as needed

9. Monitor vitamin B12, A, D, E, and K status

10. Early referral to speech and/or occupational therapist to initiate oral feedings and avoid oral aversions

11. Cycling of TPN for 2 to 4 hours daily may be attempted once the preterm infant is able to maintain blood sugars

## REFERENCES

Bianchi A. Longitudinal intestinal lengthening and tailoring: results in 20 children. *J R Soc Med* 1997; **90**:429–432.

Ching YA, Gura K, Modi B, Jaksic T. Pediatric intestinal failure: nutrition, pharmacologic, and surgical approaches. *Nutr Clin Pract* 2007; **22**:653–663.

DiBaise JK, Young RJ, Vanderhoof JA. Intestinal rehabilitation and short bowel syndrome: part 2. *Am J Gastroenterol* 2004; **99**:1823–1832.

Drenckpohl DD. Adding dietary green beans resolves the diarrhea associated with bowel surgery in neonates: a case study. *Nutr Clin Pract* 2005; **20**(6):674.

Gura KM, Lee S, Vallim C. Zhou J, et al. Safety and efficacy of a fish-oil based fat emulsion in the treatment of parenteral nutrition associated liver disease. *Pediatrics* 2008: **121**:e678–e686.

Javid PJ, Collier S, Richardson D, et al. The role of enteral nutrition in the reversal of parenteral nutrition-associated liver dysfunction in infants. *J Pediatr Surg* 2005a; **40**:1015–1018.

Javid PJ, Kim HB, Duggan CP, Jaksic T. Serial transverse enteroplasty is associated with successful short-term outcomes in infants with short bowel syndrome. *J Pediatr Surg* 2005b; **40**:1019–1023; discussion 1023–1024.

Siebert JR. Small intestinal length in infants and children. *Am J Dis Child* 1980; **134**:593–595.

Sondeimer J, Cadnapaphornchai M, Sontag M, et al. Neonatal short bowel syndrome. *J Pediatr Surg* 2006.

Vanderhoof JA. *J Pediatr Gastroenterol Nutr* 2004; **39**:S769–S771.

Wessel JJ, Kocoshis SA. Nutritional management of infants with short bowel syndrome. *Semin Perinatol* 2007; **31**:104–111.

# Chapter 27

# Summary

The goal of current nutritional recommendations is to support a growth pattern that mimics physiologic fetal growth. Are we routinely meeting that goal? Probably not, as the premature and especially the ELBW infant grows more slowly after birth if we compare them to the growth rates of normal fetuses. Certainly neonatal morbidities and inherent differences that exist between the intrauterine and the postnatal environment and metabolic conditions make this goal to mimic the fetus challenging.

One major problem that confronts all of these infants and is fundamental to growth is their nutrient intakes. This intake is often less than the support necessary to mimic fetal growth. The Lucas data relating nutrient content (protein and energy) of formula with mental and motor outcomes later in life and the NICHD Growth Observation Study linking in-hospital growth velocity with cognition, neurologic impairment, and growth outcomes at 18–22 months of age clearly demonstrate why avoidance of growth restriction is so important.

Nutrient intakes currently recommended by various international committees and expert panels are discussed in this book and are based on the concept of providing sufficient nutrients to achieve postnatal growth approximating that of a normal fetus of the same postmenstrual age. Nutritional requirements do not stop at birth. After birth, the newborn infant starts using its own glycogen and fat reserves and its protein in muscle and other organs and tissues, to maintain metabolic rate. Waiting "until the infant is stable" is incorrect because without early TPN these ELBW infants enter a catabolic condition and rapidly exhaust energy reserves. Catabolism does nothing good for the ELBW infant!

Glucose is provided intravenously at 6–8 mg/kg/min immediately after birth and adjusted to achieve and maintain concentrations between 45 and 120 mg/dL. Similarly, lipid is required to provide at least 0.5 g/kg/d to prevent essential fatty acid deficiency. Beware of providing excessive carbohydrate and lipid to the VLBW infant based on the incorrect assumption that they are necessary to promote protein growth rates. Unfortunately, even when postnatal weight growth mimics fetal growth, body composition differs from that of the fetus because of excessive fat deposition in organs such as the liver and heart as well as adipose tissue. Promoting more organ and adipose fat as well as visceral fat deposition has no benefit and causes many problems.

Amino acids in early TPN are essential not only for body growth but for metabolic signaling, protein synthesis, and protein accretion. The strategy of using insulin to promote protein growth is ineffective and further contributes to abnormal adipose tissue deposition.

A recent study from Lucas and colleagues from the same cohort of preterm infants that showed higher protein improving growth and reducing neurodevelopmental deficiencies in infancy now suggested these children as adolescents had unfavorable markers of risk for insulin resistance. It was suggested that rapid early growth in the first two weeks of life was responsible. Competing outcomes emerge from the same critical period of nutrition: a favorable effect on growth and neurodevelopment but an unfavorable effect on risk of cardiovascular disease or type 2 diabetes later in life.

Based on their studies, Lucas et al. concluded that the first two weeks of life in the preterm infant may represent a "critical growth window" during which nutrition may have its greatest beneficial and adverse effects.

Figure 27.1 illustrates that in our opinion in 2009 the benefit of early aggressive nutrition to prevent delayed brain growth and subsequent adverse neurodevelopmental outcome takes priority over the potential adverse consequences of growth acceleration in infants. However, data from the large NICHD cohort did not demonstrate growth acceleration in any of the infants and in this cohort the growth acceleration may occur later in infancy. Thus the data of Lucas and others need to be placed into proper perspective. Emphasizing protein intake with appropriate energy intakes that do not result in excessive accretion of adipose tissue may impact positively on long-term health consequences.

Early enteral feeding including the strategy of MEN is important. Ehrenkranz suggests we must overcome the biggest barriers – ourselves and NECiphobia – to ensure that minimal disruption of the transition from intrauterine to the extrauterine environment occurs when referring to early enteral nutrition strategies.

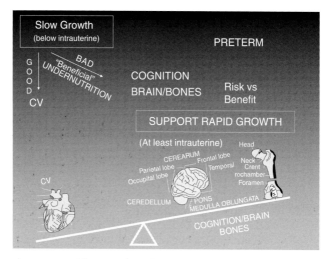

Figure 27.1 Risk versus benefit

Enteral protein feeding requirements have been reevaluated and demonstrate that fetal lean body mass gain and the contributions of protein gain to lean body mass gain are more useful than weight gain. In addition protein is necessary for early catch-up growth to compensate for the cumulative protein deficit developed in the first weeks of life. An increase in the protein/energy ratio is mandatory to improve the lean body mass accretion and to limit fat mass deposition.

Human milk plays a significant role in promoting lean body mass and avoidance of maldistribution in adipose tissue. Significant benefits to the infant's immunological sensory-neural development, gastrointestinal maturation, and aspects of nutritional status are achieved with human milk. However, the nutritional adequacy for the VLBW infant (particularly protein, calcium, the variability in nutrient content) results in unpredictable nutrient intakes for an infant who is not feeding ad libitum. As growth rates in hospital from RTBW through discharge of 18 g/kg/d are desirable, unfortified human milk will not meet the target. Reviews of multinutrient fortification of human milk studies demonstrated short-term improvements in weight gain, length, head circumference, and bone content without any difference in the development of NEC.

Emphasizing the fortification of human milk has resulted in further hypercaloric strategies for VLBW infants. VLBW infants being fluid-restricted because of lung disease have a difficult time receiving adequate protein and minerals to meet optimal nutritional requirements and growth. New products in formula development and human milk fortification make for improved nutrition even with fluid restriction.

Integrating anthropometrics and laboratory measurements is important in the management of the VLBW infant. Assessing growth and nutritional status allows for evaluation, reassessment, and intervention. Intrauterine and postnatal reference growth charts provide a base set of information at birth and offer a method to monitor growth as a measure of nutritional status. The laboratory provides the means to detect deficiencies or toxicities before clinical symptoms develop.

Growth failure in VLBW infants is common despite advances in neonatal care and the post-discharge period presents another opportunity to enhance nutrient repletion, bone mineralization, and growth. Enriched formulas that contain more protein, minerals, vitamins, and trace minerals than are contained in standard term formulas or fortified/supplemented human milk are the recommended feeding of choice in the post-discharge period.

When formula composition is considered for the VLBW infant it is important to distinguish between formula that is enriched (PDF, SSC®30) vs. formula that is concentrated (contains more energy per 100 mL). Enriched formulas contain more macro- and micronutrients than a standard formula rather than energy alone.

The neonatologist's dilemma in 2009: catch-up growth or "beneficial undernutrition" in VLBW infants. How should they grow? In a recent study of 29 term infants and 38 preterm infants ($28.8 \pm 2.1$ weeks, birthweight $1190 \pm 370$ g) at term equivalent age, the preterm infants were significantly lighter and shorter than term infants. There was no difference in fat mass as measured by magnetic resonance imaging between the two groups. The subcutaneous tissue volume was lower in the preterm infants. However, the percentage of intraabdominal adipose tissue volume was higher in the preterm than the term infants, indicating increased central adiposity in the preterm infants at term-equivalent gestational age. The authors found that increasing severity of illness had a statistically negative impact on percentage of subcutaneous tissue volume but a positive impact on visceral or intraabdominal adipose tissue volume. Perhaps it is not rapid growth that leads to increased abdominal fat mass, increased risk for cardiovascular disease, and insulin resistance later in life. Can these problems be secondary to the early increased illness severity and lower rate of weight gain? It is interesting that these findings are the same as those described two decades age when Bhatia and Rassin demonstrated that premature infants were shorter and fatter (by skin-fold methodology) than their in-utero counterparts. The care of the premature neonate is a work in progress and continues to evolve as we care for smaller and more premature infants. The care to this vulnerable group of babies makes "nutritional strategies" an integral part of the approach to ensure survival and better long-term outcome.

### SUGGESTED READING

Bhatia J, Rassin D. Uthaya S, Thomas EL, Hamilton G, et al. Altered adiposity alter extremely preterm birth. *Pediatr Res* 2005; **57**:211–215.

Ehrenkranz RA, Tounes N, Lemons JA, et al. Longitudinal growth of hospitalized very low birth weight infants. *Pediatrics* 1999; **104**:280–289.

Ehrenkranz RA. Early, aggressive nutritional management for very low birth weight infants: what is the evidence? *Semin Perinatol* 2007; **31**(2):48–55.

Kuscel CA, Harding JE. Muticomponent fortified human milk for promoting growth in preterm infants. (*Cochrane Review*). The Cochrane Library; 2005.

Lucas A, Morley R, Cole TJ. Randomized trial of early diet in preterm babies and later intelligence quotient. *BMJ* 1998; **317**:1481–1487.

Singhal A, Lucas A. Early origins of cardiovascular disease: is there a unifying hypothesis? *Lancet* 2004; **363**:1642–1645.

Singhal A, Fewtrell M, Cole TJ, et al. The impact of early nutrition in premature infants on later childhood insulin sensitivity and growth. *Pediatrics* 2006; **118**:1943–1949.

# INDEX